THE BOOK OF SHIATSU

Saul Goodman

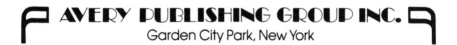

AVERY PUBLISHING GROUP INC.

Garden City Park, New York

Edited by: *Patrick M. Riley*
Cover designed by: *Rudy Shur and Martin Hochberg*
Original cover art by: *Akiko Aoyagi-Shurtleff*
Graphic Interpretation: *Susan Ure Reid*
Design and Production: *Susan Ure Reid with Sandra L. McDaniel*
Photography: *Chris John*

ISBN 0-89529-454-0

Printed in the United States of America

9 8 7 6 5 4 3 2

Contents

This book and its energy is dedicated to my father, teacher, and friend, Henry Goodman.

I would like to thank the many people who have contributed in various ways to the creation of this book.

Saul Goodman

Preface

There are many speculations as to how and when shiatsu began. Some claim that it is 5000 years old; others say that it is only 100 years old. As we begin to realize the essence of shiatsu, we realize that it is timeless. Shiatsu's origin is an outgrowth of the order of nature expressed in a fundamental human exchange. This order is simply the process of making balance, which is the primary activity of all life. In this sense shiatsu goes on mechanically in the environment, in the check and balance of the animal, vegetable, elemental and energetic worlds, and within all of the spheres of human life. It goes on within our body balances of acid and alkaline, temperature regulation, red and white blood cell maintenance, in the balancing of sugar levels, hormones, etc. It goes on within our senses, emotions and intellect, as well as socially and ideologically.

Within the environment, if this process becomes stagnated or imbalanced, nature produces an opposite stimulation to create a balancing movement. This can occur in the form of an earthquake, volcano, storm, atmospheric pressure change or temperature change. In our human life this process is also going on in order to maintain our form and function within the environment. If we become imbalanced in one way, then a stimulation for opposite movement occurs. When we become weak, for instance, a situation presents itself which engenders strength. Nature works by attraction and repulsion. What comes to us or goes away from us is a result of the condition we consciously or unconsciously produce by our way of life. This movement and shifting to make balance can manifest in a myriad of ways. It appears in the realm of health, in varying degrees, as colds, flu, kidney stones, cancer, etc. It appears in daily life circumstances in the form of romance, relationships, monetary success or failure, injury or accident. Basically, however, these forms all represent the transition of energy to make harmony which is the constitution of our universe.

As human beings we enjoy the unique quality of making a choice in how we create these balances. The development of our judgement is simply the refinement of deciding and creating our choices rather than being subject in our lives to the effect of unconscious choice.

The art of shiatsu, practiced to create a balance of our energy, is an innate part of being human. It employs the use of our hands as an extension of our heart and as an expression of our compassion. Because this ability is so commonly based everyone has the ability to give effective shiatsu. Experience in teaching has found this to be true. Shiatsu connects us with something essential to life and is primary to the development of our health and happiness. We intend this manual to assist everyone in bringing forth their shiatsu.

Author's Note

The Shiatsu Practitioner's Manual presents a synthesis of traditional oriental techniques, adaptations for the Westerner's mode of learning, and elements which encourage shiatsu to evolve as an art form. It presents what I am calling the 'Nervous System Response' which is based on the function of the autonomic nervous system, and has developed from the need in teaching to bridge the sensitivity and wisdom of the Far East with the technological mind of the West.

In approaching all areas of expression — art, science, architecture, horticulture, business, etc., Orientals begin from an inbred, intuitive, natural understanding that the universe is generated from an unlimited 'source' which endlessly produces *ki* energy. 'Ki,' which is sometimes translated as 'life force,' condenses to appear as all aspects of our manifested world. In contrast, Western culture has developed with the material and structural plane as its starting frame of reference. This presents certain challenges in studying arts originating in the Far East, as the Western student has little or no experience in perceiving the world as 'ki.'

The autonomic nervous system and its response offers a unique device for bridging the differential of East/West perception. While it has been well studied as a physiologic system and anatomical structure, at the same time, the obvious function of the nervous system is to receive energy and vibrational impulses from the environment and to distribute them throughout the body and mind. The nervous system also gathers the energetic product of body/mind activity and transmits it back out to the different strata of our environment.

The study of the autonomic nervous system serves another purpose of this manual. This is to clarify that all aspects of our human experience, from physical to spiritual, are activities of well-defined systems of energy. The more physical systems, such as circulation and respiration, are easier to identify whereas the more invisible systems, such as the world of emotions, are only perceivable through higher senses which develop quite naturally through practices like yoga, meditation and shiatsu. This multitude of systems, which serve as different functions of energy, interchanges and interacts to form the whole of our internal and external universe. The study of the autonomic nervous system and its two branches also demonstrates the universal paradox of two seemingly opposite forces making harmony. The parasympathetic branch describes the absolute world and the sense of the 'whole'. The orthosympathetic branch and all of its responses describes the relative world and the 'parts' of the whole.

I have further chosen to present this study of the autonomic nervous system as an example of the universal scheme because of its direct use and compatibility with learning shiatsu. By practically understanding how the skin responds to touch and how these responses are triggered by the nervous system, we can more easily sense and monitor changes in the more subtle energy systems.

Another theme threaded throughout the text comes from the experience I have had from teaching and giving shiatsu. This is the realization that, as the times have changed, so has the meaning and application of this beautiful art form of human expression. Giving shiatsu has taught me the intimate connection between touch and our entire human experience. The clinical applications of shiatsu, mostly developed and collated in China and Japan, are already well studied and documented. In this manual I hope to expand the meaning and use of shiatsu as a tool for personal and societal transformation.

The effect of giving and receiving shiatsu has deep penetrating effects on ourselves, friends, clients and environment. In the future I would like to incorporate its use in the natural education of our children and as a lay healing tool within the family. Humanity itself is another functioning energy system within the environment and the condition of balance within this system affects the whole of nature. Now, in this time, while the 'system' of humanity desperately seeks harmony, the simple exercise and widespread use of one of our most natural qualities, or shiatsu, is essential.

Saul Goodman.

Introduction

Shiatsu Goes West

Over the past fifty years healing methods of Eastern and traditional origin have found their way into our Western society. Natural treatments such as acupuncture, herbology, moxabustion, and the use of medicinal foods are now finding acceptance and being used regularly in the United States and Europe. Among these practices, shiatsu massage stands out as one of the most practical, simple, yet effective methods.

Shiatsu, traditionally translated, means finger or thumb pressure. This implies that the practitioner, by applying pressure to another person's body, effects various responses and changes in the body's functions. In actual practice a variety of pounding, stretching, rocking and manipulation techniques are used. Pressure may also be applied by use of the forearms, elbows, palms, feet, and knees.

After a shiatsu treatment the recipient may feel lighter, more balanced, and enjoy a sense of calmness. The body functions more smoothly and the person feels revitalized. Many times sleep is deeper and more restful; therefore a person's overall requirements for sleep can be reduced. Symptoms such as stiffness, headaches, sluggishness, and backaches often disappear, while clarity and quickness of thinking tend to improve. Conditions related to reproductive problems, structural misalignments, and emotional difficulties often improve with shiatsu as it assists the body's primary systems and functions in re-establishing their normal rate of balance and activity.

How Shiatsu Works

Shiatsu is based on the premise that body and mind, which operate as one, are created by, maintained by, and work by energy.* Energy circulates throughout the body along well-defined passageways called *meridians*. Along the meridians are points called *tsubo*, which translates to mean: 'Where the cycling of electromagnetic energy gathers.' A tsubo might be compared to a volcano, where energy deep within the earth's core rises to the surface and is released. Likewise, tsubos are places where energy is particularly active and interchang-

---

*Energy in oriental medicine is called *ki* or *chi*. It is often translated as *life force*. These terms are used interchangeably throughout the text.

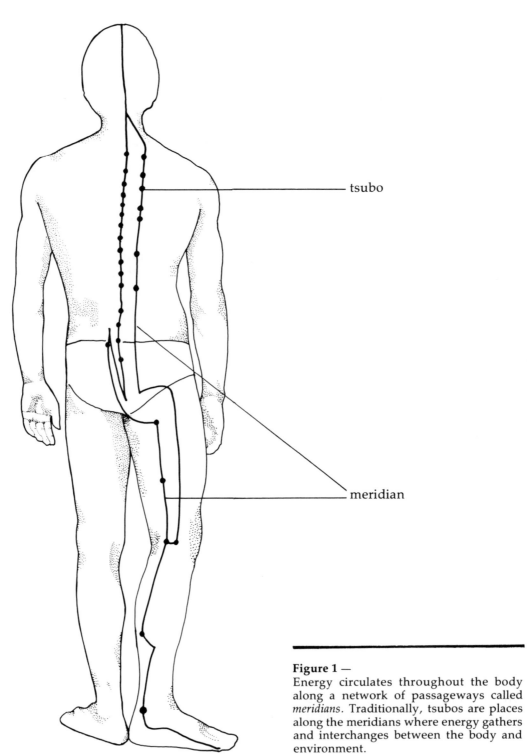

tsubo

meridian

Figure 1 —
Energy circulates throughout the body
along a network of passageways called
meridians. Traditionally, tsubos are places
along the meridians where energy gathers
and interchanges between the body and
environment.

ing with the environment. In shiatsu, tsubos are experienced with a dimension of breadth, depth, and response to the practitioner's touch. In the more technical practice of acupuncture, tsubos are located in very specific places along a set of traditional meridians. (See Fig. 1)

In shiatsu the meridians can be extended and tsubos can be anywhere on the body. This is possible in that the body as a whole is a manifestation of energy and because applying pressure anywhere on the skin surface will affect the body's multiple energy systems. Scientific research has demonstrated that the meridians and tsubos are intimately connected with the body organs and life systems. It has been established that these energies, in proper supply, are vital to the workings of all body functions.

When an unbalanced condition develops in a body organ or system, it is transferred to the surface through related meridians, tsubos, and branches of the nervous system. This can appear in correlated areas as pain, stiffness, roughness, change in temperature, or discoloration of the skin. It can also create numbness or loss in mobility of the extremities. These symptoms, though commonly viewed as inconvenient and usually dealt with through symptomatic approaches, are actually valuable signals or warnings of stagnation and imbalance occurring within the body. Through the various techniques of manipulation, a stimulating or governing effect can be relayed back to the troubled organ or system. The techniques used to create stimulation are called *tonification*, while those used to diminish energy are called *sedation*. These influences, when applied to the related meridians, points, or areas, help to reorganize the total body energy field, creating balance. Hence the ailing condition and its symptoms will subside or disappear.

The traditional wholistic approach is that irregularities in body-mind function are a consequence of a person's way of living; this means the sum total of their thinking, eating, personal habits and perspective on life's circumstances. Although shiatsu treatment can re-establish energy balance, if the person continues to pursue the lifestyle responsible for causing poor health, the tendency to develop the same or deeper problems in the future will remain. On the other hand, if the person is willing to change these detrimental habits, shiatsu can be a tremendous catalyst to improving and creating good health.

After treatment, the practitioner will often offer further suggestions that are helpful in promoting sound health, and in preventing a possible recurrence of the original problem. These recommendations are based on his or her knowledge and experience of how the body works and on what affects its well-being. This can include dietary advice and way of life suggestions as well as corrective exercises for reinforcing the benefits of the treatment. In keeping with the spirit of all traditional natural healing methods, the person is encouraged to discover for himself the cause and meaning of his own problems.

Ancient Meets Modern (or East Meets West)

The introduction of shiatsu and acupuncture to the Western world was met with skepticism by the scientific and medical communities. The concept of meridians connecting the body, and of invisible energies which could not be detected by any type of meter or graph, seemed quite far-fetched. This reception reinforced the modern status quo in that if you cannot see it, touch it, or measure it, it cannot be real (even if you can feel it!). The idea that a problem area of the body could be treated locally as well as through manipulation of distant points connected to it by invisible energy networks seemed impossible. It was hard to believe that conditions such as constipation, ringing in the ears, paralysis, tooth pain, etc., could be treated by external points along the arms, hands, legs, and feet. Anesthesia without drugs; treating left side pain by manipulating the exact opposite place on the right side; increasing blood circulation and respiratory rate by the laying on of hands — these things were considered just 'unscientific'.

This pinpoints the essential difference between the modern Western view of life and the traditional ancient view. Within modern Western thinking the person is seen as a separate entity from nature and the parts of the body and its functions are studied as separate. Traditionalists view the person as integrated with the total environment, and understand the interconnection of the internal and external, the biological and the environmental. This makes for a more complete, in-context evaluation of a problem, its cause, treatment and cure. For example, when a person develops a knee problem, contemporary therapy only investigates the anatomy and mechanics of the knee. The condition of the cartilage is examined for degeneration, weakness and strength of the tendons and ligaments are tested; positions of the bones are checked. If fluid has developed, it is removed and checked for volume and the presence of blood. Often a progression of treatments varying in degrees of severity and cost will follow. These can range from casts and external applications to internal injections or ingestion of cortisone, steroids, and pain-killers — treatments that carry with them the possibility of long-term weakening as well as side effects and damage to the rest of the organism. If pain, injury, discoloration, swelling or degeneration continue, more extreme replacement procedures with artificial, synthetic, biologically disconnected parts are used. Meanwhile the cause of these symptoms remains mysteriously unknown, unexplained and unaccounted for.

The wholistic traditional way is to discover the cause of injury, weakness, degeneration, and even accident by reviewing the whole person and his way of life. It looks for the internal organ or function that may be troubled, causing distress to arise at the knee or in other related body areas.* The person's skin color, tone of voice, body odor, and outward expressions are all taken into account. Dietary habits are a focal point as food directly creates and influences

---

*See Part 7 — Diagnosis

the body's energy, organ function, and development of blood quality. Usually simple manipulation and dietary change based on understanding this whole picture will remedy the situation. Symptoms generally adjust and disappear smoothly as the person regains normal health and strength without much physical, emotional, or financial stress, and without permanent disability.

Later in time, when dramatic results from these wholistic methods were evident, the critics began to concede, "Well, it seems to work." However the contention was and still is being held; "But we do not and cannot know why." What we must realize is that we can know how these methods work, especially if our modern society is ever to lift itself from the dilemma and destruction created by its present technology. Thousands of years ago these methods were developed around the common knowledge and understanding of energy and how it is the origin of man and nature. These understandings are available to us through a sixth sense called intuition, around which ancient people based their whole lifestyle. Modern thinking overlooks and tends to completely invalidate intuition as superstitious and unscientific. Ancient peoples, on the other hand, discovered and developed many advanced technologies in the practice of healing, architecture, agriculture and science by using these intuitive understandings.

A Hand With Our Development

Shiatsu has many unique aspects. Unlike other forms of treatment it requires no specialized knowledge or years of memorizing technical data. There is no need for special equipment, machines or tools such as needles, knives or x-ray. The shiatsu practitioner makes use of man's simplest, basic tool: his hands. Use of the hands is one of the main qualities that make man unique. Through the dexterity of the thumb, which structurally marks a turning point in human biological evolution, man can bring forth the physical counterpart of his imagination and thoughts. The creation of civilization, its architecture, technology, and arts, began as man developed the ability to translate his mental images into physical reality.

How we use our hands shows what is in our hearts. In terms of energy, the heart represents the balancing center or *chakra**, between the base physical energies of the sacrum and abdomen, which are connected with intuition, and the mental consciousness center of the mid-brain.

---

*Chakras are key energy centers in the body which are connected to various physical, emotional, psychological, life expression and spiritual qualities. Human beings have seven.

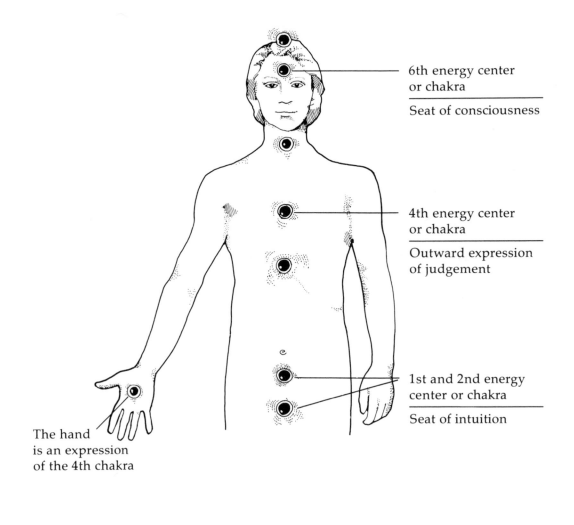

6th energy center
or chakra

Seat of consciousness

4th energy center
or chakra

Outward expression
of judgement

1st and 2nd energy
center or chakra

Seat of intuition

The hand
is an expression
of the 4th chakra

Figure 2 — Chakras are key energy centers in the body which are connected to various physical, emotional, psychological life expressions and spiritual qualities. Human beings have seven chakras.

The hands, by energy and function, are extensions of the heart and help us to outwardly express the sum total of our intuition and consciousness, or what could be called judgement.

We can see that human development and expression coincide with the ability to use the hands, especially the thumb. Man, being a creature of higher consciousness and spiritual awareness, is also able to communicate on a more refined wavelength. So by expressing ourselves through the hands and developing their use, we further create our human spiritual quality.

Continuity of Life

Recently it has been discovered that not only is all organic life (animal, vegetable, virus, protein, fungus, etc.) completely interrelated and totally dependent on the assimilation, use and constant discharge of energy, but that the inorganic worlds of elements, atoms, protons, neutrons and electrons share the same relationships. Without these invisible energies no physicalized phenomena would exist. They are a complete backdrop to the material world. To support this a special technique of photography, called Kirlian photography, which is capable of recording and making these energies visible, has now been developed.

Now twentieth-century man is discovering what was common understanding in the ancient world. One wonders why our modern schools refer to our ancestors as primitive and uncivilized. In its real sense "primitive" means those that understand the balance and harmony of nature and base their thought, expression and way of life upon it. Real shiatsu is like this. It is an expression of making balance, the basic activity of nature. It is approaching life with deep respect and acknowledging that all humans and animals, as well as the vegetable world, elemental world and energy spheres, are related and interdependent. It is acknowledging that making balance is common and essential to all life.

2

Energy Has Order

Energy Has Order

In its search for order and harmony our society has become progressively more aware of the world of energy and its integrated relationship with all the facets of our day to day living. This awareness has worked its way into our modern lives, appearing in everything from slang expressions to the continuing studies of science. Energy has become a household word which many people now use to express themselves, often without consciously connecting it with the actual mechanism they are describing. Comments such as: "My energy is low"; "They have good energy"; "I'm going to put my energy into it," have become commonplace. Recently, in movies, people and moving objects have often been portrayed with vibrations of energy surrounding or trailing them.

After a thousand years of developing theories and concepts around the belief that energy and matter are separate, the sciences have now returned to investigate and substantiate the ancient beliefs that the two exist as one. The study of quantum physics has demonstrated that physical phenomena are appearances of energy in different stages of activity. The walls and floors around us, the food we eat, and the clothes on our backs are nothing but energy in condensed, materialized form. In studying waves of energy interchanging with minute subatomic particles of matter, researchers have found that the wave and particle, which seem to be separate, are actually conditions of the same phenomenon.

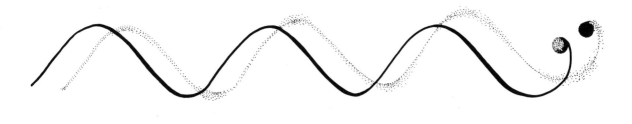

Figure 3 — Wave and Particle.
The wave and particle phenomenon studied in subatomic research presents the basic paradox of energy and matter. If viewed from a perspective of energy, this activity appears to have speed and movement. If seen from a perspective of matter, it appears as a particle occupying a particular pattern.

When measuring the speed of waves scientists discovered that they lost or were unable to determine the position of the particle. When identifying the position of the particle they could not gauge the speed of the wave as it seemed to disappear. This demonstrated that the separation of the two was an illusion of the senses. The wave and particle were both the same thing at the same time. In an attempt to find the smallest building blocks of matter, science discovered that this physical world exists as a form of energy. After identifying atomic, sub-atomic, and preatomic particles as the smallest components of matter, researchers discovered that it was actually energy and vibration that were the building materials of the physical world. It was realized that matter in different ratios of time always returns to the realm of energy, and that all phenomena and their movements manifest in a wave-particle appearance.

The illusion of energy and matter is similar to a ceiling fan which, when spinning, appears to be a solid disc. In actuality it is only individual blades revolving at high speed.

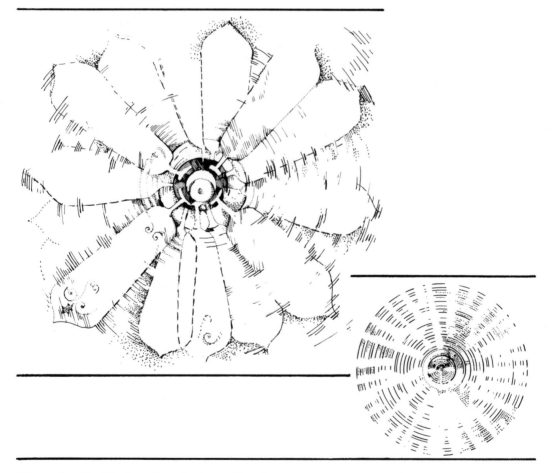

Figure 4 — The illusion of a spinning ceiling fan.

How we relate to the world through the conditioned perception of our senses is analogous to the experience of seeing a tree bending by the power of the wind. We point and say "It's the wind." Really we cannot see the wind; what we are observing is the result of an invisible force. In a similar way, the physical world we perceive through our ordinary senses is a result of the movement of energy and only appears to be solid and static. This principle applies from the largest galaxy to all aspects of our human body and its functions, down to the smallest micro-organism and non-organic particles.

In discovering how the energetic world intermeshes with the physical world, physicists also found that the laws of physical matter did not seem to apply to the realm of energy. It appeared to them that, for the most part, energy and its more primitive manifestations of preatomic activity moved at random and in no apparent order.

However, if we put a piece of paper on top of a magnet and pour iron filings on top of the paper they will arrange themselves, due to the magnetic energy field, in patterns of definite order.

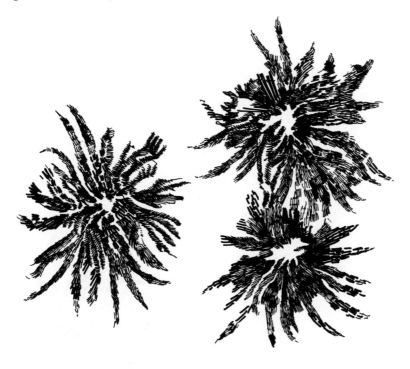

Figure 5 — Iron filings arranged around a magnetic field.

In the same way this world is arranged around a very definite pattern of energy which also moves with a well-defined order. The universal spirallic pattern can be observed everywhere in nature. It appears in the structure of the

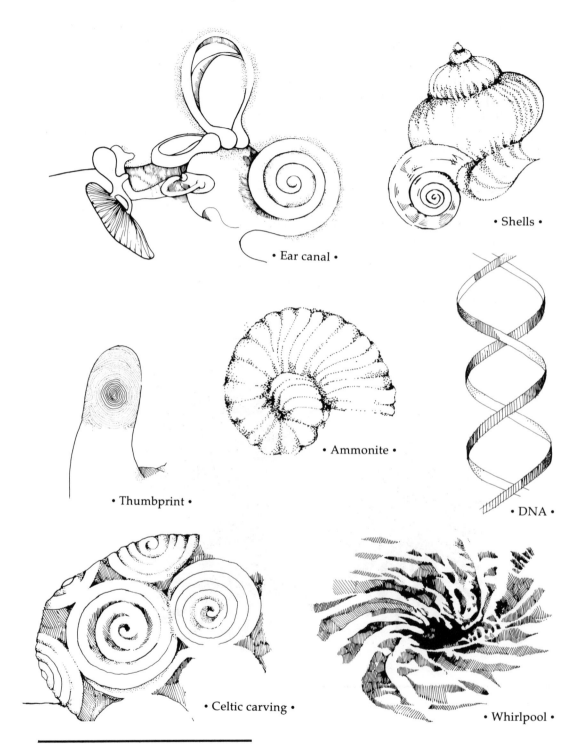

• Ear canal •

• Shells •

• Thumbprint •

• Ammonite •

• DNA •

• Celtic carving •

• Whirlpool •

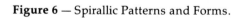

Figure 6 — Spirallic Patterns and Forms.

galaxies, solar systems and their movements; in the progression of weather and ocean current movements; and in the overall make-up of all life forms. It appears in the hair spiral, in the formation of the ear canal, in our fingerprints, in DNA, and in the overall structure of our bodies. We can even observe the spiral in the movement of water going down the drain.

The spirallic pattern itself results from the interaction of two primary energy movements. These movements are *centripetal*, contracting tendency and *centrifugal*, expanding tendency. These two forces appear from what both philosophy and science have identified as an endless, unlimited, generating source which connects, propels, sustains and diffuses everything in this universe. Throughout time, this source has been mutually identified by all writings, philosophies, and religions under different labels such as Infinity, Oneness, God, the Almighty, and so on. Now, even modern science is on the verge of confirming this collective ancient understanding.

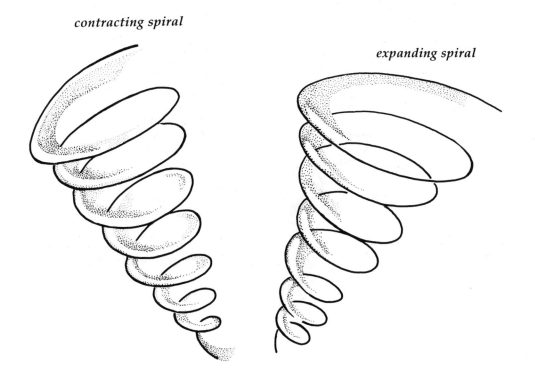

Figure 7 — Spirallic patterns of contraction and expansion arising from an endless, generating source.

The centripetal tendency of energy we refer to as *yang* (△) or *Heaven's force*, because its direction and generating point is coming from the outer environment in towards the earth. The centrifugal tendency of energy is *yin* (▽) or *Earth's force* because it generates from the earth outwards. The understanding and application of these two complementary yet opposite forces, and the spiral which they cooperatively produce, appears constantly as the cornerstone of ancient civilizations and is evident in their works of art, medicine, sciences, philosophies, religions, and cultures.

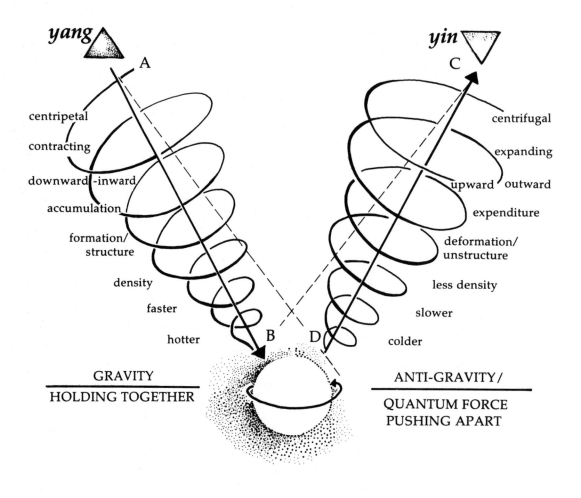

Figure 8 — A-B is the course of materialization influencing energy to appear physically. D-C is the course of spiritualization influencing energy to appear in the form of vibrations. B and D are the transition points.

Since the time of Newton, scientists have identified gravity as an energy that seems to be pressing down on the earth, exerting a force which holds things together. More recently, a force which moves upwards in the environment has been identified as anti-gravity. Researchers have also recognized this tendency which works against the force which holds things together, that is one that seems to push things apart. They call this quantum force. So modern physicists have now essentially discovered yin and yang, although they have yet to fully appreciate the dynamic relationship inherent in these terms. They have yet to see the wealth of applications of this unique principle already available within ancient technology, health practices and sciences.

Heaven's force, or yang, is more obvious as it manifests seven times more strongly than Earth's force, or yin. This ratio of 7:1 appears in our modern environment in, for example, the width and height of an ocean wave, the ratio of head to body in our human structure, and the power ratio of the heart's left chamber (7) to right chamber (1). Escape velocity is another example in that a rocket must accelerate to seven times the force of gravity in order to be able to leave the earth's atmosphere.

This basic order is the orientation of nature. All phenomena move according to this vacillating cycle of expansion and contraction. Most phenomena, if we take the time to look, can easily be seen in this context of motion, rhythm and order; others are moving too quickly or slowly to observe. We can say that the former lie within our usual parameters of perception, while the latter lie outside this boundary.

As we develop our awareness of these universal cycles of expansion and contraction, our parameters begin to expand until we eventually see all things from this largest, or what we could call *macrobiotic* viewpoint.

The most immediate and easy way to see this order of nature is in the cycle and rhythm of the heart which is expanding and contracting every second within our body. At an extreme of expansion and taking in blood the heart contracts, pumping blood out. The lung cycle has a slightly slower rhythm of 3-5 seconds, taking in oxygen on expansion, and releasing carbon dioxide on contraction.

The digestive tract is in a state of constant motion. This facilitates the absorption and conversion of our foodstuffs in a cycle which takes from two to four-and-a-half hours. Under the influence of our vacillating body conditions, our thoughts, emotions, and behavior go through cycles of change and perception in time periods which range from seconds to periods of days and months. The environment also undergoes perceivable cycles of expansion and contraction. Each day has an orderly pattern of change reflected in our routines of daily living. We experience cycles of biorhythm every 23, 28 and 33 days, and women of course experience a very complex revolution of menstruation every month. As we become more in tune with these processes, we can eventually see multiple rhythms unfolding in the course of our entire lives.

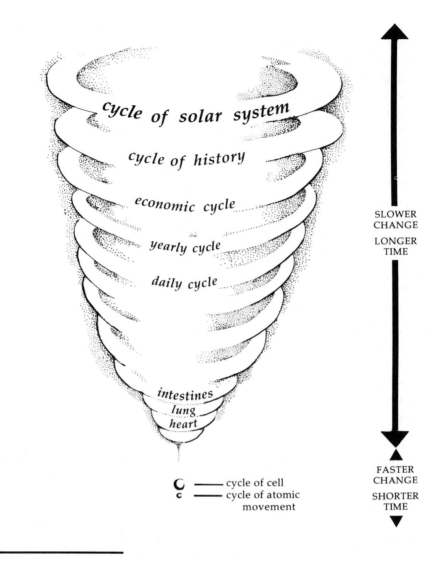

Figure 9 — Cycles of Change.

Beyond the limits of our ordinary perception, moving too slowly for most people to detect, are the expanding and contracting cycles of economics occurring every 12, 18, 60, and 120 years. History itself, if plotted in a logarithmic spiral, assumes the same alternating form as does the rotation of the solar system around the galaxy which occurs every 200 million years. Moving much too quickly for our average senses to perceive are the cycles of cellular activity, and changing even more quickly is the world of preatomic particles. (Figure 9)

Studying nature through the eyes of yin and yang is the most simple and direct way to understand our lives and the world around us. By being aware of these forces as the basic motivation in all the constant change that we experience internally and externally, we can uncover the mysteries of everything from the common cold to cancer, science, human physiology, dietary balance, relationships, and any other conceivable area of research.

Yin and Yang Relationships

yang	*yin*
hotter	colder
center	periphery
more dense	less dense
organ	meridian
animal	vegetable
day	night
male	female
mineral	protein, fat
more dry	more wet
faster	slower
material	spiritual
structured	free form, diffused
horizontal	vertical
aggressive	passive

Figure 10 — Yin Yang relationships.

The Five Transitions of Cycling Energy

While going through phases of expansion ($\bigtriangledown$) and contraction ($\triangle$) all phenomena pass through five discernible phases. The study of these five phases, which became the focal point of Oriental medicine, is called *Go-Gyo* or the *Five Transformations*. The five phases, each with its own distinctive quality, are called *Fire, Soil, Metal, Water,* and *Wood (Tree)* respectively.

The most active or expanded part of the cycle is likened to the energy of fire and is represented in our body by the heart and small intestine and their respective qualities.* As the energy of contraction becomes dominant it creates a stage of gathering, downward and inward motion like the energy of soil. This stage is represented in the body by the spleen/pancreas and stomach and their

*See Part 7 — Five Transformation Diagnosis for the extended qualities of the organs and meridians.

qualities. Reaching the extreme of contraction, energy appears consolidated or like metal. It is represented in our bodies by the lungs and large intestine. Highly condensed energy begins to relax and open, as the yang dominance transfers to yin dominance. This stage is like water and is represented in the body by the kidneys/bladder and sexual organs. Energy then rises in the cycle and begins to move outward in a dispersing motion. This energy is like wood or a tree and is represented in the body by the liver and gallbladder. Energy then reaches its most active, dispersed stage and the cycle begins again.

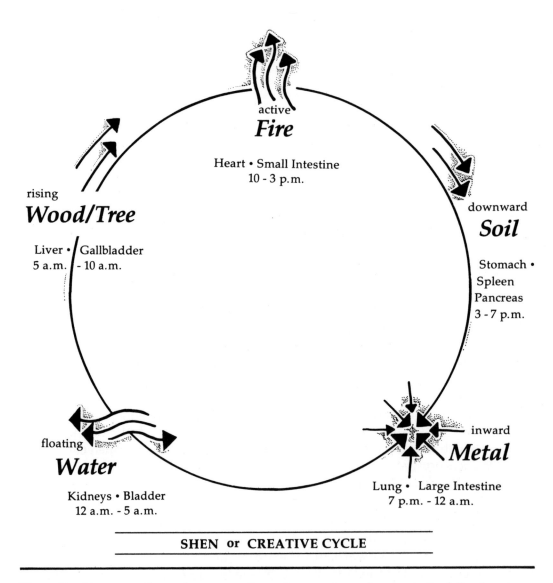

active
Fire

Heart • Small Intestine
10 - 3 p.m.

rising
Wood/Tree

Liver • Gallbladder
5 a.m. - 10 a.m.

downward
Soil

Stomach •
Spleen
Pancreas
3 - 7 p.m.

floating
Water

Kidneys • Bladder
12 a.m. - 5 a.m.

inward
Metal

Lung • Large Intestine
7 p.m. - 12 a.m.

SHEN or CREATIVE CYCLE

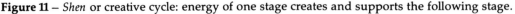

Figure 11 – *Shen* or creative cycle: energy of one stage creates and supports the following stage.

Each stage has a particular quality of energy which then generates and creates the quality of the next. This is called the *shen,* or *supporting* cycle, and is similar to the relationship of a parent and child. On the other hand, (See Fig.12) if we overstimulate the activity or tendency of any stage in the cycle, it creates a suppressive or antagonizing effect on the stage of opposite nature. If we overactivate rising, wood/tree energy, it inhibits or aggravates the gathering, soil part of the cycle. If we stimulate the active, fire part of the cycle, it inhibits the consolidating, metal stage of the cycle. If we stimulate gathering or soil energy, it

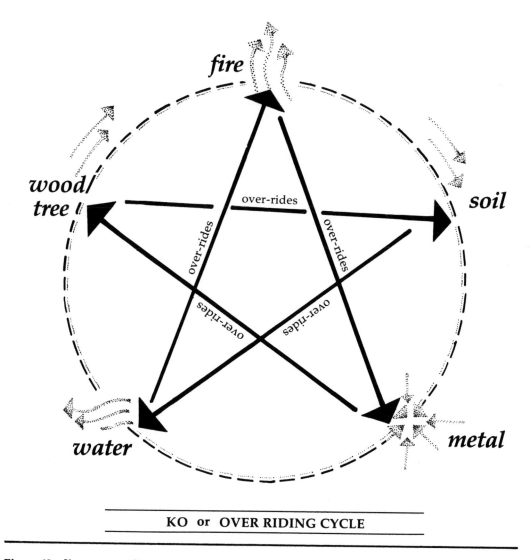

KO or OVER RIDING CYCLE

Figure 12– *Ko* or over-riding cycle: energy of one stage inhibits or suppresses the movement of an opposite stage.

interferes with relaxing, or water energy. Stimulating metal, consolidating energy inhibits the rising of tree energy. Stimulating floating or water energy makes the active, fire stage slow down. This is called the *ko* or *over-riding* cycle.

The stages of energy transition during day and night are a good example of the supporting-creative, *shen* cycle. The morning, between 5 a.m. and 10 a.m., is generated by rising or wood/tree energy. Most people are influenced by this charge as they get up and move outwards for their daily activities. Between 10 a.m. and 3 p.m. is the most energetically active time of day correlating with the fire stage. At this time people are most busy performing their daily tasks. Telephones are busier, the stock markets are active, construction is going on, and cars, trains, and buses are at the peak of moving to various destinations. From 3 p.m. to 7 p.m. soil energy is most active. People focus on going home as rush hour traffic reflects energy directed in a determined, yang way. Between 7 p.m. and midnight people gather in homes and public places as activities reflect the more inward inclination of metal energy. From 12 a.m. to 5 a.m. energy develops into a floating phase. People are generally quieter and resting.

The Five Transformations are used in a very detailed way in the practice of acupuncture and Chinese medicine. In the study of shiatsu they can be used in a more generalized way for diagnosis. We can also utilize our observation of these transforming energies as a means of recognizing the endless unfolding of energy and as a vehicle to seeing the order in which energy continuously appears and changes.

3

The Nervous System Response

Overcoming the Biggest Barrier

One of the biggest challenges for students in beginning the practice of shiatsu appears when they are introduced to the study of invisible energy systems, chakras, and auras. This happens because seeing and working with these mediums lies generally beyond the range of their current experience. Even though they may for the most part agree that these energies can exist and function, it still seems overall like a remote, intangible concept and leaves them feeling confused, uncertain, and groping in the dark.

On the other hand most of us are masters of sensory perception and physical sensation. In other words, if we feel hot or cold, we are absolutely confident in what we have experienced. Even when we go to touch hot water or an ice cube we can anticipate what it will feel like before we make contact. We can also easily judge weight, color, light, wetness, etc. If someone slaps, squeezes or caresses us, we know what these sensations are and can distinguish them in their many degrees of intensity. Human beings are, in fact, capable of a very sophisticated and well-rounded differentiation of physical sensory perception which our intellect and experience allow us to compare and arrange into infinite categories.

Energies which are generally inaccessible to the five senses, such as meridian ki flow, chakras, and aura can also be detected, judged, and compared. To do this we must develop the 'non-mind' sense of intuition, which becomes available to us through our practice of shiatsu, along with self development exercises such as do-in, yoga, breathing and meditation. As it takes time to develop and trust the sense of intuition, frustration often arises when learning and practicing shiatsu, which deals directly with diagnosing, treating, and influencing these invisible energy systems. Therefore what we need to discover and use is an intermediary connection between the sensory level and the nonsensory, invisible level. I have found that the bridge between the detectable and undetectable is our nervous system.

Any stimulation that comes within range of our senses is immediately picked up and relayed by the nervous system complexes to the brain for interpretation.

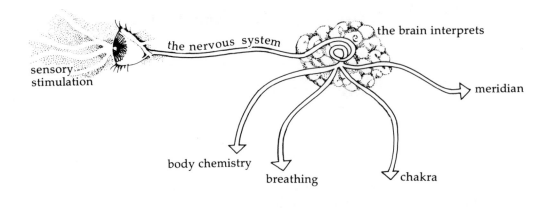

Figure 13 — Sensory stimulation causes reaction and adaptation by all the body and energy processes.

Other spheres of function and energy, such as breathing and meridians, simultaneously react, adapt and adjust. At the same time invisible waves and images are constantly received by the energy networks and are translated via the nervous system to the physical body, creating adjustments on the level of cellular activity, blood fluid chemistry and hormones, as well as structural alignment. (See Fig. 14).

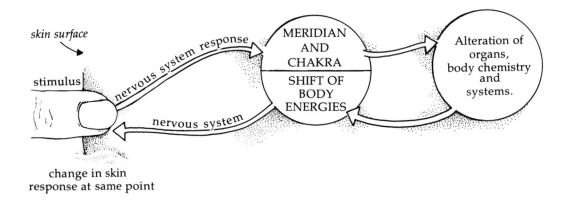

Figure 15 — Circuit of Change. Stimulus to the skin surface causes a chain reaction of change, adaptation and alteration of all physical and energetic systems. These shifts of quality and activity are relayed back, creating a perceivable change in the response of the skin surface.

When shiatsu is given, stimulation at the skin surface triggers a response of the nervous system. This effects a reaction and change in the meridians and chakras. Together these changes create adjustments of the body chemistry, systems and organs. The changing, adjusting meridian and chakra energy conversely influences the nervous system which in turn alters the skin's response to the stimulus. (Fig. 15)

This adaptation mechanism of the skin, called the Nervous System Response, helps us monitor changes occurring in the invisible systems as translated back via the nervous system. With practice and concentration we can feel and interpret these changes which have many variations and occur with different degrees of intensity. (See Part 5. Preliminary Exercises).

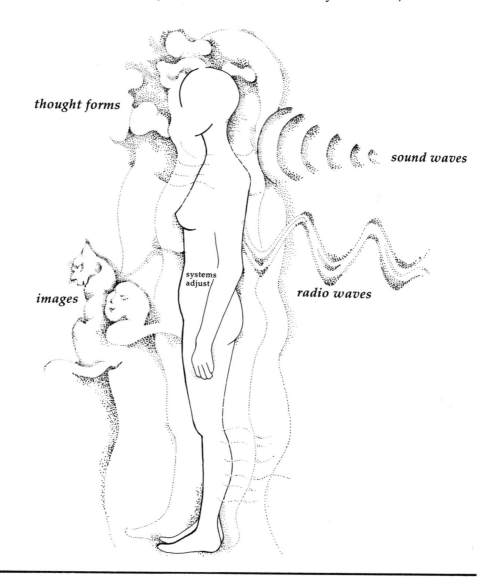

Figure 14 — Invisible waves, thought forms and subliminal images are received by the energy systems and interpreted to the body processes via the nervous system.

The conscious and accurate gauging of this response is an excellent starting point for realistically working with energy flows, and lies well within everyone's range of ability. Although this ability takes time and experience to develop, it will eventually lead the practitioner to a more intuitive level of interpreting, affecting, and anticipating the reactions of the receiver's energies.

The Autonomic Nervous System and Energy Response

The nervous system has a conscious part that responds to our commands and an unconscious part, called the *autonomic nervous system*, which coordinates, triggers and conducts all of the involuntary functions of the body. The autonomic nervous system itself has two branches which are opposite yet complementary in the effect they have on our mind and body function. These branches are the *orthosympathetic (ortho)* and *parasympathetic (para)* systems. Our perceptions on all levels of experience change completely depending on which branch is more active.

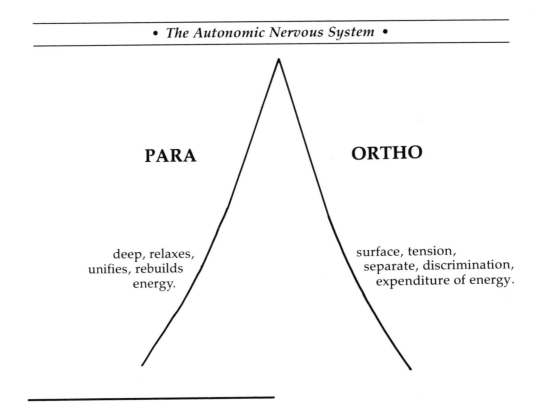

• *The Autonomic Nervous System* •

PARA

ORTHO

deep, relaxes, unifies, rebuilds energy.

surface, tension, separate, discrimination, expenditure of energy.

Figure 16 — The Autonomic Nervous System.

The orthosympathetic system or mode is connected more to the surface of the body and its activity relates to separation and discrimination of distinct sensory perceptions, along with responses of tension. When this branch is more active, body and meridian energies are more distinguished and specified in function. Ortho also tends to influence expenditure and dissipation of energy. The parasympathetic system or mode is more involved with the deep body processes, and its activation provides a unifying experience of body, mind, spirit and environment.* When para is more active, energies tend to merge, balance, regenerate and function as a whole. (Fig. 16). The para and ortho modes of perception can be compared and related to what researchers have identified as left and right brain phenomena.

The ortho mode which initially picks up any stimulus we receive, isolates and identifies it as a separate sensation.

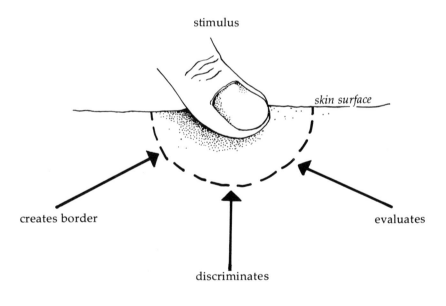

Figure 17 — ORTHO tenses; the body isolates and scrutinizes stimulus. The receiver is consciously aware of a single point: resistance.

---

*Reference to para generally implies a balance in the overall autonomic nervous system, with a slight dominance of energy charging the parasympathetic branch. Although ortho can dominate in a balanced condition, it tends to overdominate in most unbalanced conditions.

Once this system, which is related to the body's defense mechanism or 'fight or flight' response, is satisfied that the stimulus is not potentially harmful to the survival of the organism, its activity diminishes and recedes. The effect of the stimulus will then be transmitted by the para mode which allows it to be experienced beyond the point of contact and eventually by the whole body. Therefore when the activation of ortho recedes, the sensation at the point of contact is integrated into the body's entire system and experienced via the para system.*

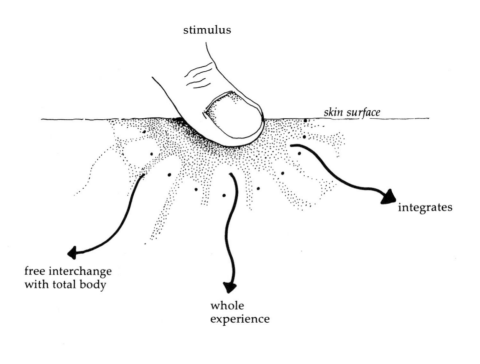

Figure 18 — PARA relaxes (ORTHO goes into background). Stimulation diffuses throughout the body. The receiver becomes unconscious of individual point.

We can get a feeling for how the body energy works in accord with the autonomic nervous system by comparing it to the lock system of a canal. When we feel relaxed due to a more dominant para mode, energy begins to flow freely, encouraging excesses of energy in one area or meridian to dissipate while deficient places regenerate. The body and all its deep life processes are balanced and revitalized. This is similar to when the locks of a canal open, letting water

---

*See Preliminary Exercises, kyo-jitsu, 1, 2, 3, Part 5, page 59.

flow between the sections, thus balancing the water levels and allowing the movement of a vessel between the locks.

ORTHOSYMPATHETIC MODE:

Energy is more specified to a system, body area, or meridian. In an extreme condition of stimulation to this system, energy starts to become locked.

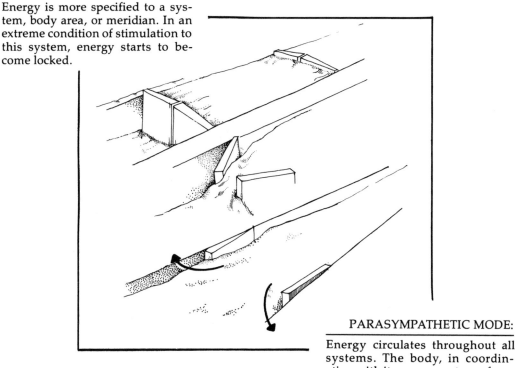

PARASYMPATHETIC MODE:

Energy circulates throughout all systems. The body, in coordination with its energy systems, functions as a whole unit.

Figure 19 — Canal Locks.

When the ortho mode is actively dominating in a state of tension, it resembles when the locks are closed. Water remains separated by the lock and movement between sections is prohibited. Similarly, body energy is being specifically dispatched to one or several particular functions or areas. A good example of ortho control is what often happens when driving a car. As we drive, especially in heavy traffic or for long periods of time, the heart speeds up and breathing becomes shallow; adrenalin continuously pumps which tightens the kidneys and lower back muscles. This syndrome is further activated as these reactions then cause more energy to go to the ortho system.

If the stimulus we give during shiatsu treatment is too strong or is applied too fast or forcefully, the surface or ortho sense stays active, creating protection and tension. Stimulus, if gradually applied, allows the body to adapt and accept it, and encourages the ortho response to recede and then give way. The point of contact then integrates with the whole body energy as the stimulus is picked up and relayed by the para system.

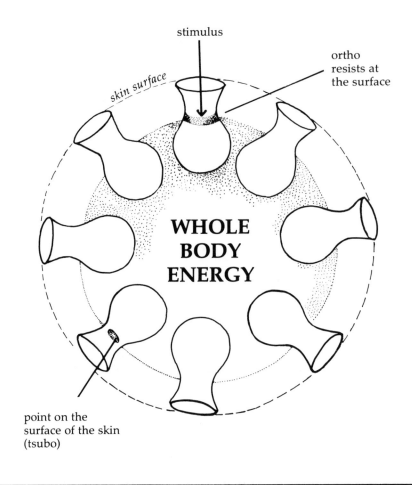

Figure 20 — (i) ORTHO holds the impact of the stimulus at the surface while evaluating its potential effect.

Points that are weak and deficient in energy are more defensive, they resist longer to changing and adapting to the stimulus. If we approach these places by patiently holding them, the protective mechanism eventually gives way allowing us to sink more deeply to the bottom of the point*.

---

*This sinking to the bottom of the point may be only a fraction of an inch.

This creates two noticeable results. First, the whole body is then receiving the stimulus. Second, by connecting this point with the whole body energy system, the point is then nourished and revitalized by an influx of energy.

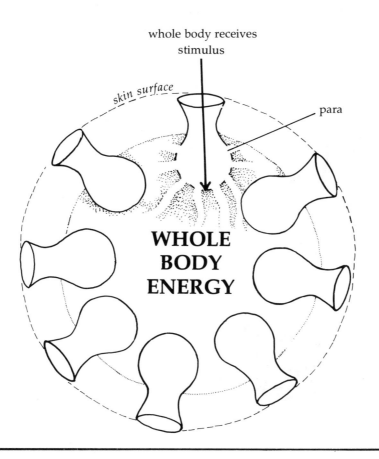

Figure 20 — (ii) PARA allows the effect of the stimulus to integrate with the whole body energy.

There is a definite change in sensation that the practitioner can feel as these changes take place. This requires focus and careful attention to what is being felt under the hands. As your sensitivity increases you will begin to feel a subtle electrical-type charge in each point and along the meridian. If the point is already charged you will anticipate and feel it immediately or within seconds of contact. If the point is empty, you need to wait patiently and hold with pressure until the shift of sensation takes place and energy comes. Eventually, by your intuitive sense of energy you will bypass the places that are already charged, and spend more time holding and influencing the weak, inactive ones.

Getting the receiver to experience an open, unified state of energy is the primary goal of the method presented in this manual. Once the whole body relaxes and energy is freely moving through the various systems, more specific balances and alignments are made available to us through working with specific points, meridians, muscles and manipulations. It is like opening the door to a

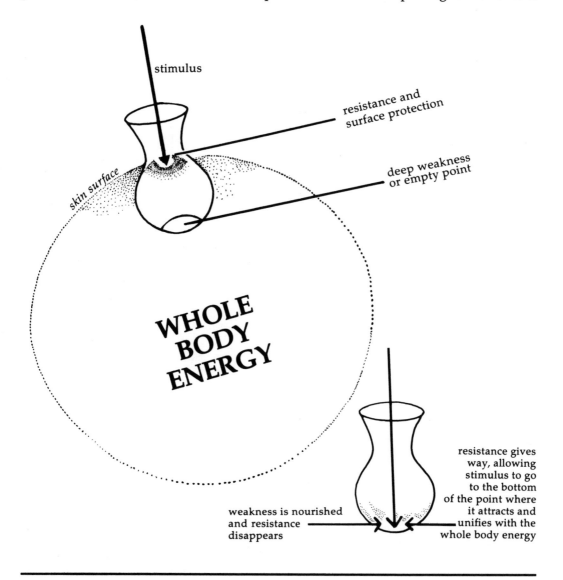

Figure 21 —

house. Once we enter we can move freely about the rooms, rearranging them or changing their appearance if we wish. *In shiatsu, getting the receiver to relax, open, and trust our touch is the initial step in treatment.* Assisting the reorganization of energy is the second step and can only be done if the first is accomplished.

When we study the body and its relationship to the environment, we discover that its form and function, including the meridian system, are products of environmental order. In a sense we are directly plugged into nature via our energy system. This means that the energy system, nervous system, blood and hormone system etc., react to and interchange with weather patterns, ion changes, planetary and constellation movements. When the environment changes on any level from social circumstances to natural phenomena, such as a drop in the barometric pressure, our complete energy field adapts to make balance. Physically, emotionally, and psychologically we are immediately influenced. Even our judgement, actions and decisions can be altered.

There are orderly ways in which to see and study the changes and influences of the natural environment. Even though they are not included in this manual, awareness of them can be helpful for our practice. The more conscious we become of these changes, the more effectively we can interpret our condition and that of the people around us.

When we are in a state of ortho dominance the body closes and withdraws from these external relationships. When we are relaxed and open, the energy systems move freely and interchange with the external influences from which they originated and evolved. Therefore many balances and normalizations of the systems will automatically occur. So, even though the primary stage of treatment is preparatory, it can of itself effect deep and dramatic changes.

Summary

Sensing the shift from ortho to para mode tells us several important things:
1) The overall condition of energy at the point of contact.
2) That the energy meridian system has changed.
3) That the point of contact has been integrated and nourished by the whole body energy.

If the shift does not occur or is delayed, this tells us that:
1) The point has remained closed at the surface.
2) The body is protecting the area of contact at the surface.
3) The point is separate energetically from the total body function. This also relates to the condition of whatever the point is connected to, such as organs, nerves, muscles, systems, etc.
4) The body as a whole is closed, protecting weakness.

4

Spirit Attitude and Dimensions of Shiatsu

A general and simple shiatsu treatment can be very powerful and effective. On the other hand a complex, technical approach can be useless, leaving the recipient feeling disoriented, bored and wondering what its purpose was. Overall, what does decide the quality and effectiveness of our treatment?

With everything we do in this life, the most important ingredient is the spirit with which it is done. Spirit is formed from the transformation of the energies of our experiences. Consciously directing our spirit creates enthusiasm and results in a complete participation in the present.

$$SPIRIT = \frac{experience}{energy} \left.\vphantom{\frac{\frac{experience}{energy}}{\frac{spirit}{conscious\ direction}}}\right\} IN\ THE\ MOMENT$$

$$ENTHUSIASM = \frac{spirit}{conscious\ direction}$$

So along with developing the natural technique of shiatsu, we need to discover the spirit behind that technique which allows the technique to emerge. It is the same spirit we need to discover and exercise in order to fully experience, benefit and grow in any activity of life. Spirit, which is formed by the consciously directed movement of energy vibration, is common to everything we do.

When we become solely focused on technique or results, our activities become mechanical and lifeless. When we utilize techniques and enjoy the process of their use as a vehicle for the expression of spirit, then what we are doing, regardless of what it is called, gives us a feeling of being alive, happy, and light. Whether we are driving a cab, waiting on tables in a restaurant, supervising a construction site, teaching school, or giving shiatsu, we always have the opportunity to develop and express our spirit for life. Any occupation, hobby, or activity that we consciously or unconsciously choose to pursue provides a format of experience within which to realize our most basic human needs and expressions. Each situation, when we examine the multiple facets it has to offer, makes the meeting of these needs available in a way that perfectly complements our present level of growth.

For some, coming to the study of shiatsu may be a catalyst for progressing and growing within some other endeavor. This is one of many possibilities. Others may stay with shiatsu for a long term or a lifetime, using it as a context within which to develop themselves. Through learning and developing our understanding of shiatsu, we begin to see its likeness to all of life's activities in that it deals with the movement, transfer and transformation of energy. As we begin to practice we also see that shiatsu inherently offers a very direct way of realizing the experience we are actually seeking by taking part in any other type of job, hobby, project or expression. Therefore, by practicing shiatsu, we enhance and deepen the experience of our life's activities. Likewise, by exercising our spirit through enthusiasm in anything we do, we can develop our shiatsu ability.

The immediate reasons for being attracted to finding out about shiatsu are many. For some it may be curiosity while others are not sure and just 'have a feeling.' Some attend a workshop because it appears to offer a way to change occupation or develop a career. Some are seeking to relieve chronic symptoms while others want to learn shiatsu as an adjunct to other body therapy. Many of these initial responses are superficial reasons that lie at the surface of our motivation. They unconsciously mask deeper seated needs.

Newcomers to shiatsu often sense that it offers an experience they are seeking in order to change and enhance their lives. Beckoning them forward this study appears as a way to develop awareness and self-expression. Like the tip of an iceberg all of these initial reasons are easily seen, yet in reality are a very small part of something much larger yet invisible.

We have this vehicle we receive upon entering this life called bodymind. This is our ship or vessel in which we travel the ocean of life and have the experience of human being, or being human. This is what, in the beginning stages of growth, we call 'self' or 'I'. In the course of many experiences we spot the tip of this 'shiatsu iceberg.'(Fig. 22)

Initially we are attracted to shiatsu as a way of making changes or as a new and different way to improve our lives. It may appear for instance as a more enlightened way to survive and make money. Then when we discover what is underlying these initial attractions and see the many dimensions of shiatsu practice, we realize that it is an innate human characteristic we all eventually express in some way, through some means, at some time in the awakening of our consciousness.

Recent polls show that about 85-90 percent of the people in countries with high standards of living do not enjoy, look forward to, or get fulfillment from their daily work. That is why they are putting reset buttons on alarm clocks which most people hit three to four times every morning. Our contemporary society, with its emphasis on technology, leaves most people dissatisfied in their day-to-day activities. Something seems to be missing. The directed spirit of enthusiasm, which determines our liveliness, and the enjoyment of the step-by-step means of achieving our ends, are totally overlooked by our results-oriented culture. So now people are feeling empty. They are seeking some spark to reintroduce vitality into their aspirations. As a by-product of this desire, they are attracted to activities that encourage well-being through a positive, wholistic approach to life.

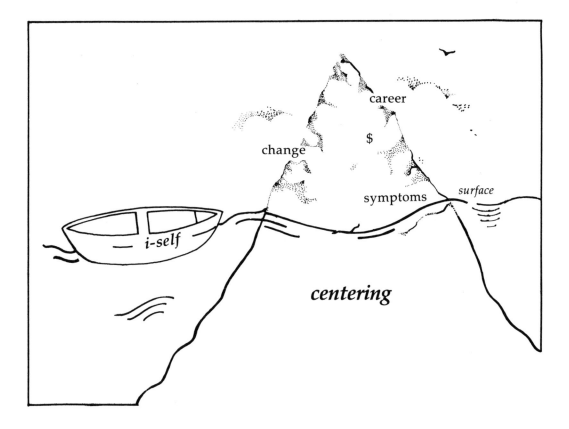

Figure 22 — Shiatsu Iceberg.

The first stage in beginning our practice is to realize why we have consciously or unconsciously chosen to explore shiatsu. The connection is no coincidence. It is a result of our basic human need and desire to fully experience life by consciously shaping and bringing forth its circumstances. Through our ongoing shiatsu program we have discovered the following qualities to be the larger invisible reasons for which people are knowingly or unknowingly interested in learning about shiatsu. At the same time they are the inherent properties of shiatsu upon which its success and effectiveness depend.

Centering

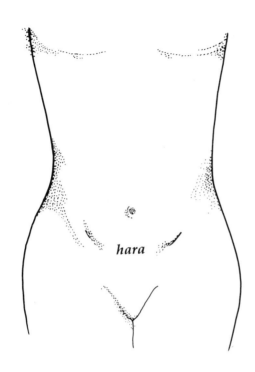

In the 'new' or 'Aquarian' age, many centering practices are becoming popular. These are developmental exercises and disciplines which enable us to focus our energies in and strengthen our physical center. This physical center (see Fig. 2) is called *hara*, the very center of which is called *tanden*. Centering techniques such as meditation, martial arts, yoga, and breathing encourage the body energy to become balanced. Through focusing energy in the hara, the mind, emotions and spirit become united and our actions and reactions harmonize appropriately with the natural and immediate environments.

Figure 23 — Hara

The proper practice of shiatsu initiates automatic centering as it is essential that all our movements and techniques originate from the hara. When moving from the hara, energy focuses there with several effects on the practitioner:

1. We begin to develop centered body movements.
2. We activate the function of intuition and begin to develop this sense and its use.
3. By acting from intuition, we can easily make harmony with the receiver's needs by the use of our technique.

Acquiring the quality of centeredness within the practice of shiatsu has an added dimension. Whereas many practices focus on 'self centering,' shiatsu extends the experience the practitioner is having outwards to others, opening up the initial stages for sharing and giving. These qualities then begin to consciously manifest within all activities, enriching the experience of our individual and collective lives. (See Fig. 24.)

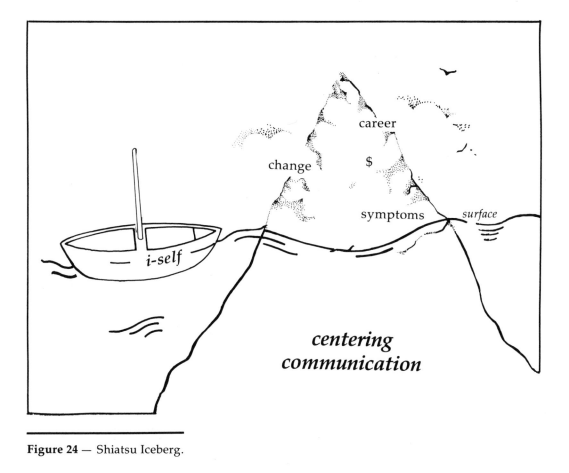

Figure 24 — Shiatsu Iceberg.

Communication

In its contemporary usage many people may be confused and misled as to the meaning and experience of communication. It is generally thought of and taught as a process where something is spoken by one person and received as a message by another person who then gives an appropriate answer. Basically the first person directs thoughts or ideas verbally at a second person who then returns a trained or automatic response. This approach actually sets up and perpetuates a separation, fostering an emphasis on and restriction within individuality. The word individuality itself means 'in dividing' or 'making duality'. It allows us to remain insensitive to and unconscious of what is really being conveyed. When we begin from a context where we put ourselves outside or apart from others, we can get lost in an illusion of separation. This sets the stage for expectation, blame and delusion in our relationships, and for misunderstanding in our human affairs overall.

In order to give someone shiatsu, we need to have empathy for what that person feels. We must be able to experience what it is like to be in their body and to have their mind. While giving treatment we are asking ourselves, "Where is their pain, emptiness, sorrow? Where is their joy, strength and aspiration? What is their life experience?" We need to feel these things as if they were our own. Then automatically our body and hands will begin to move in a way that gives this person relief. Our touch becomes sensitive and compassionate to their wanting and they feel nourished as our shiatsu encourages a balancing of their various energies. In giving true shiatsu, we create an environment of real communication. If we explore more deeply, we find that communication involves much more than verbal exchange. It contains a broader level of expression in the form of feelings, images, actions and reactions. Much more transpires on this subliminal level, beneath the exchange of words, through the interaction of our more refined energy systems. These systems, particularly the meridians and chakras, reflect and carry the influence of all our past and present experiences and expressions. The progressively more dense systems of psychological, intellectual, emotional and sensory energies integrate and then embody the more refined energies and their influences within the physical posture.

This network of interchanging energies provides the most direct and primary channels of communication and occurs within a larger framework of vibration within which we all co-exist. In developing our shiatsu, we develop our sensitivity, awareness and involvement in this deeper level of exchange. We do this in the most basic way: through centering and touch, which opens up and releases the movement, flow, and interchange of energies. When we touch someone in shiatsu, it releases these energies which contain forms, images, feelings and past experiences, many of which may have been locked in the various systems. It is on this level of energetic exchange and through these mediums that we express our more personal inhibitions, evaluations, desires, and needs.

The word communication itself contains the root 'commune' attached to the ending 'ication' meaning action or motion. Commune or communion means 'becoming one'. In giving shiatsu, we develop our sense of oneness. In time, as we practice, we begin to realize and experience a higher connection with all of the many worlds around us. This connection then becomes the root of our perception and expression in everyday life.

A sense of oneness or connection is another aspect missing and overlooked in our modern approach to life. The problem this creates is obvious when we view the tenure of present day human relations, in family, community, business, and on a global scale. Many people, through various methods, are now seeking this ingredient in their lives, although the majority go about looking for what seems to be an elusive element, without being able to clearly identify it. In essence this unifying fabric, this universal connection that we become aware of through true communication, is the real nature and expression of love. It is not only what we commonly seek in this life, it is at the same time the unfolding of what we really are.

In giving shiatsu, we develop this sense of real communication by experiencing the other person's body, mind and life as a natural integrated part of treatment. (Fig. 25)

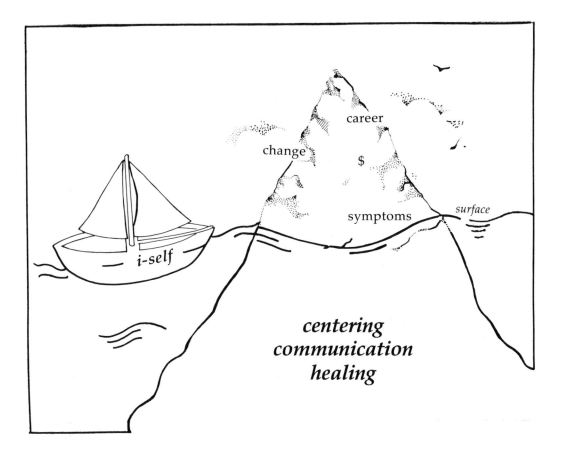

Figure 25 — Shiatsu Iceberg.

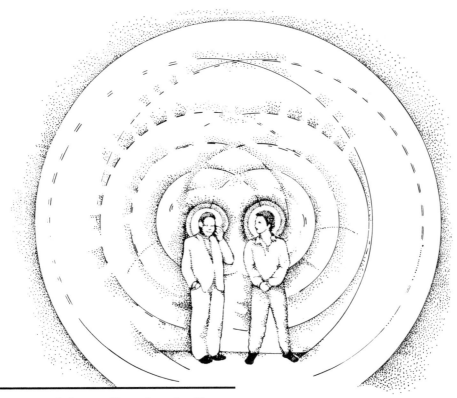

Figure 26 — Spheres of Interchanging Energy.

Figure 26 — There are many spheres of circulating, interchanging energy which make up the whole of our being. Each sphere has its own quality, character, vibrational frequency, and density. The uniqueness of a sphere is what we identify as body organs, systems, emotions, mind, etc. Although they can appear to operate separately, they are constantly interchanging, and eventually diffuse into larger, more refined, less personalized fields of energy. The transfer of our energies or what we eventually identify as communication occurs most immediately through the refined networks which merge at different levels within the environment.

The effects or messages of this exchange are assimilated into the more dense systems which react and respond according to their respective function. If the movement of a sphere is clogged due to imbalance or stagnated vibration, the reception becomes incomplete and inaccurate in its interpretation. At the same time, the normal perception on the physical plane is to see ourselves as separate and other people and their actions as outside of ourselves. These factors can lead to unconscious conflict as the oneness experienced on the refined levels is not accurately conveyed to the more dense levels. This conflict is then perceived and interpreted in such ways as lying, deceit, covering up, excuses, etc. as the lower vibration of our words does not ring true with that of our more refined, comprehensive energies.

In one sense, the laying on of hands completes the circuit of energy on the physical level. In another sense the effect that shiatsu creates opens up the flows and exchanges between all levels of energy, giving the experience of union within and between the giver, the receiver and the environment.

Healing

When we become aware of the need to heal ourselves it often appears as a barrier or an enemy we are confronted by and need to conquer. When we become involved in this 'battle' most of us are waiting to heal our weak intestines, our anger, emotional difficulties or relationships before we can enjoy and fully experience our lives. We are struggling with the concept of becoming healed as if it were a terminal project with a definite ending point that releases us into a state of happiness and perfection. We do this similarly to the way in which we wrestle with the so-called 'difficulties' and 'suffering' in our day to day life. So, what does healing really mean?

The state of being 'healed' does not really exist. It is an endless journey that has many stages, although the basic mechanism is the same on every level. Let us take a basic physical example. When someone cuts their finger, what is actually happening? A separation is being created. Then, in the process of healing on the most basic level, two becomes one. Similarly, real healing is a continuum that permeates all spheres of our life and development. Through it we progressively develop the sense and experience of becoming one. We begin to realize and harmonize our body, mind and being with the multiple environments of social, financial, natural, and spiritual existence.

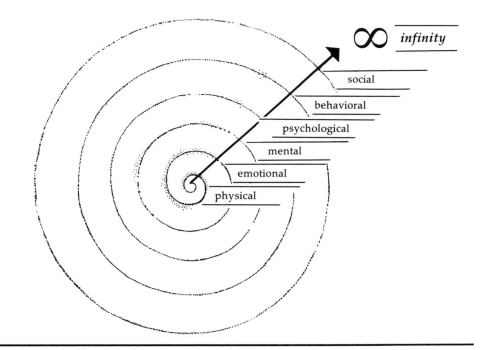

Figure 27 — Healing is a spirallic continuum through which we merge with our higher, more expanded self.

There are three stages of healing:

Personal

In this initial stage we begin to realize our imbalances in the form of sickness or weakness primarily on the physical, sensory, and emotional levels. We focus our attention mostly on ourselves and can often become consumed by these problems. Energetically many of these physical difficulties are related to the lower centers or chakras which also create our identity, ego, and concern for individuality.

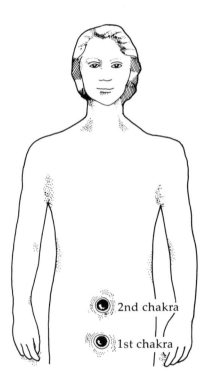

2nd chakra

1st chakra

	Physical Relationships	*Personality Functions*
1st Chakra	function of bladder parasympathetic nervous system, lower colon, gonads, reproductive function.	identity, ego, grounding material sense.
2nd Chakra	kidneys, intestines, ovaries menstruation, blood formation	confidence, creativity centeredness, sexuality

Figure 28 —

As a consequence of being overly focused on healing the functions related to these centers, we tend to continuously create their unbalanced qualities of arrogance, separation, and magnified self-concern. We are unaware that these attitudes are the real, underlying cause of the sicknesses and problems we experience in life. We therefore create a secondary barrier to truly changing our condition.

At first this level seems difficult and inconvenient in that it confronts and identifies some of our basic habits in lifestyle and diet as the creators of our sicknesses. Many times people will drop out of or avoid involvement in healing, choosing to allow the illness to go deeper and thus to degenerate by remaining attached to the causal factors.

Those of us who continue to pursue healing, grapple in this initial stage with the surfacing awareness that we are responsible for all our difficulties, and have produced them by creating personal separation from nature. During this period we may experience large emotional swings as we try to adjust our view of blame towards others and outside circumstance, to one of self-reflection.

Service

In the second stage, we begin to have the desire to help other people. We want to tell them about the methods and techniques we are using to improve our health and happiness. Initially we feel as though we are doing something for others and should be appreciated for our efforts. Often we feel let down when these people, who are themselves just entering the first stage of healing, are so overly self-concerned that they do not seem to sufficiently compensate or appreciate our endeavors.

Soon however, we begin to appreciate the experience of these interchanges when we see, as if looking in a mirror, our own egocentric, self-gratifying attitudes. We realize that on deeper levels these attitudes or mind-sets perpetuate a separation syndrome that manifests in all areas of our lives, and that this relates particularly to our persistent physical and emotional stagnations. We begin to see the resistance we have to letting go of the concepts, expressions, reactions, and habits that create a continuous lack of harmony within our own lives. Through this we gradually realize that to serve is in and of itself a healing experience and that this opportunity alone is enough of a return for our effort. As with the gift of life itself, nature has already provided the compensation for something we have yet to do. Service to others is the doorway to healing, especially of our emotional and conceptual discrepancies with the environment. It provides a bridge to the deeper experience of being unified with our surroundings. By seeing ourselves through others, we develop a compassion and empathy for the experience they are having in the journey of healing. Compassion adjusts and balances our emotions while empathy helps to dissolve our rigid concepts and broaden our intellect. We begin to recognize our sameness with others and to progressively relinquish attachment to being only individual. In the latter part of this stage we receive deep fulfillment from this work and begin to orient our lives to service.

Surrender

This third stage is the doorway to real social healing. We begin to distinguish the more immediate needs of our environment, and to realize that nature works in balance so we can embrace and respond to every situation. It becomes clear that all people and situations have multiple characteristics and that the 'front' side we initially focus on, whether it appears good or bad, weak or strong etc., has an equal, opposite back. All phenomena have this nature, without exception. When we understand clearly that the front (beauty, strength or charm) is produced by and depends on the equally opposite back (ugliness, weakness, or arrogance), we can then know that accepting both sides together as one is the only true possibility in really expressing our love. So this level serves as a vehicle to realizing acceptance and expressing love. It also leads to ideological healing. We realize that nature is produced by opposite or seemingly antagonistic qualities that must coexist and which are therefore, paradoxically, complementary. Degenerative illness, for example, is antagonistically becoming the plague of modern man while its complement is that it allows us to discover and change the discrepancies of our modern life.

Through this view, our actions and life-orientation are always in accord with the welfare and happiness of all of our human friends. We begin to understand that we truly exist as one and that our likenesses must be realized before our individual expression and interpretation can be brought forth harmoniously. Fundamental characteristics such as human structure, metabolism, blood pH, and nervous system development are prerequisites of being human. We all have the same body organs and systems although they vary in size, strength, dimension, and capacity. We are all products of a highly organized and cooperative organism. We all share the same direction in that the unfolding of our potential is achieved through the development of our consciousness. This consciousness is ultimately universal and is at the same time facilitated by our personal and mutual experience.

$$FREEDOM \ = \ \frac{Acceptance}{Surrender} \ = LOVE$$

Once we realize the true meaning of healing, we are no longer preoccupied with our weak intestines or tight kidneys although we are still aware of this physical level and continue to care for its health. Our lifestyle, which is now more deeply balanced, manifests on the physical and emotional levels, enabling them to function more smoothly. We realize that healing is the natural process of human development and potential, and that wherever we are operating within its evolution we can totally enjoy, experience and participate. We realize that we are always in a state of perfection and that happiness is this awareness.

In the practice of shiatsu we are healing ourselves through centering and communication and we are serving through sharing that experience with those to whom we give shiatsu.

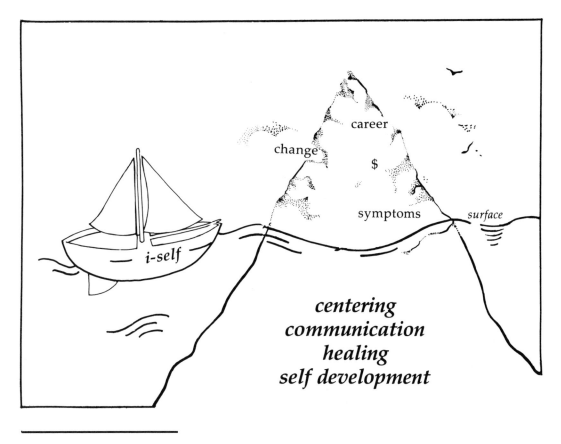

Figure 29 — Shiatsu Iceberg.

Self-Development

Self-development is the product of centering, communication, and healing, and is the prime motivation for all our actions. This self-development does not only mean our smaller immediate self, although it is included. It does not refer to the 'John Doe' or 'Mary Jane' in that we become smarter, craftier, more powerful or more talented, although these things may appear. Through true self-development we realize a sense of connection with nature as a whole, and that this entire universe actually exists as our true self. The illusion of separation that we experience throughout many of the initial stages of our development begins to dissolve. In each gradual stage we submit to the consciousness and function of our true, larger self and operate within the human plane from that orientation. This progression of growth, which dissolves our smaller, separate ego, is similar to a tributary merging with a river and then the river merging with the ocean. In order to grow we must give way to cooperation within a larger context. Whether or not we resist or deny this as our deeper purpose we must eventually discover this universal direction and embrace it. The resistance and denial of growth and expansion is itself the ultimate cause of sickness and unhappiness.

We can begin shiatsu just for the benefit of those things above the surface which are like the tip of an iceberg. If we keep practicing we will begin to realize what is underneath the surface and what shiatsu offers. If we become conscious of why we bought this book, changed our eating, breathing or thinking, we discover that realizing this true Self is what we really want to do.

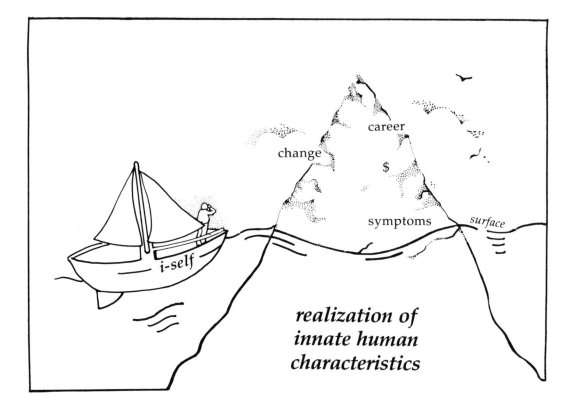

Figure 30 — Underlying the pursuit and accomplishment of any occupation, hobby or expression, is the real, innate need to realize our true self.

A Word About Shiatsu

Words which compose our various languages are created from similar sounds. Sound is a manifestation of energy and is therefore an embodiment of spirit.

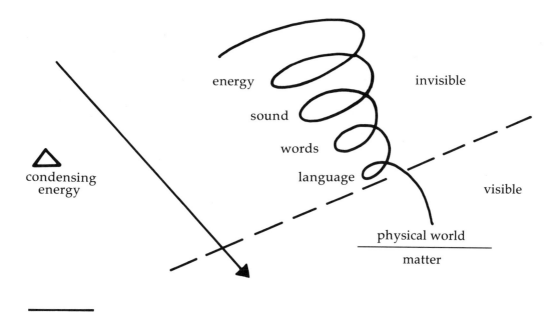

Figure 31 —

When we are speaking, the sounds which we use as words are transferring and directing energy. Our use of language conveys our spirit and can have creative or destructive effects on our multiple environments. Just as matter is an appearance of energy, sound, which also precedes matter, is a constitutional component of all physical phenomena. Within each tree, rock or mountain, certain tones are vibrating. Even the planets and solar system are generating sounds. Each of our body organs and systems relates and responds to a particular sound or sounds. This is why the practice of chanting can have regenerating, healing benefits.

Ancient and contemporary languages have two distinct qualities. Ancient words not only identify physical phenomena, they also portray their intrinsic spirit and unity within the whole process of the environment. This is why they often require several explanations in translation. These languages and their more pure composition of sound have the effect of moving energy and creating a sense of aliveness.

Conversely the modern use of language tends to focus on separating through analysis and concentration on physical quantitative aspects. Many of the words have a stagnating effect on energy, creating a heavy feeling in the environment. Words such as 'but', 'not', 'because', etc., can have an inhibiting effect on energetic flow. A phrase like 'What's the matter?' literally refers to blocked and out-of-balance energy in situations and in physical conditions. Gender and personal pronouns (I, you, they, etc.) give a built-in separating quality to the modern use of language which is nonexistent in ancient use. From the energy and spirit conveyed by the word *shiatsu* we can see how and why its practice is a very direct way to develop and realize our human potential.

Shi means thumb and, as mentioned earlier, the development of this appendage coincides with a turning point in the evolution of our consciousness. *Shi* also represents the heart which is our central organ, and relates to fire. In order to exist as humans we need to have a constantly burning internal fire of 98.6 degrees. If our temperature vacillates too high or low we begin to feel strange and our senses, thinking, and perceptions become distorted.

Shi also means plasma and is the actual nature of consciousness. Our thinking, imagery and immediate vibration are organized energy in a state called plasma. Up until thirty years ago, modern science only recognized four states of matter: gas, liquid, solidification and gross matter. Recently a fifth state of matter or plasma was discovered. Plasma appears as gas decomposes (a yin process) into the most basic components of matter which are free-streaming, unattached electrons. In this condition the electrons can either recondense into solid-like matter or dissolve into pure vibration or spirit. By discovering the world of plasma, science revealed the bridge between the spiritual and material worlds.

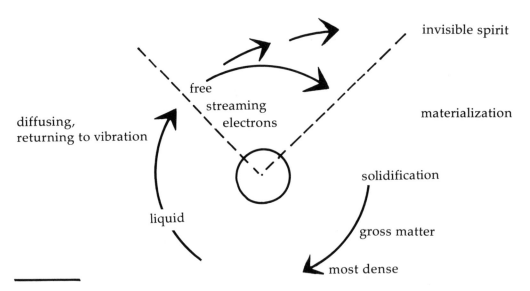

Figure 32 —

Shi also refers to the astral realm and to the composition of our astral body.

Tsu, or centripetal formation, means pressure which is the condensing of energy. *Tsu* also represents the 'cycling of electro-magnetic energy', which is the component of our immediate life force. Pressure contains these electro-magnetic energy fields and both together create our human appearance.

A connects and coordinates *shi* and *tsu*. It is sound initiating the manifestation of our will, larger self or universe into its totally condensed replica, the smaller self.

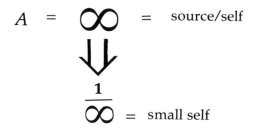

Figure 33 —

So shiatsu is a condition by which human life exists and a mechanism by which it manifests. When we give *shi-a-tsu* we are creating these conditions and addressing the basic qualities of being alive in human form.

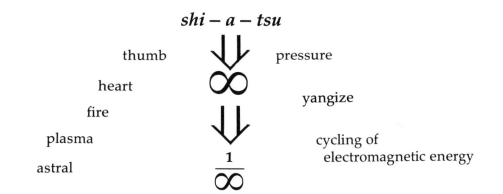

Figure 34 —

5

Preliminary Exercises

Hara

Anatomically the hara is our entire abdomen. Structurally it is our center of gravity. About 2½ inches below the navel is the center of the hara, or what is called *tanden*.

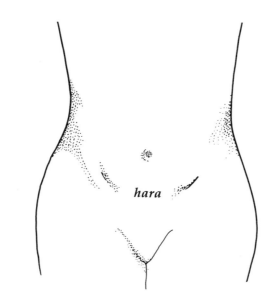

hara

Figure 35 — Hara.

To properly apply any technique in giving shiatsu we must become aware of our hara and of how all energy, emotion and physical movement is formed and generated out from it. Techniques such as giving pressure, stretching and kneading, etc., need to become extensions of the hara movement.

Our initial assessments need to be interpreted through focusing our energy in the hara and not in the mind. If we try to decide conditions of energy by our intellect alone, we can never make an accurate evaluation. If we interpret from the hara, however, then the appropriate answer becomes clear. When we allow the hara to lead, all our actions and techniques are accurate, according to the requirement of the situation; when we become centered and open we are then able to generate limitless energy. We therefore never experience tiredness or fatigue.

The following exercises are to develop awareness of hara-focused movement.

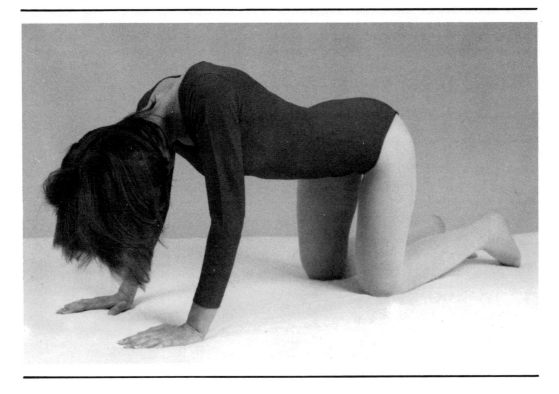

—————— **Exercise 1** ——————

Shifting the Body Weight from Hara

1 Assume the position on all fours. Find a place that feels very comfortable as if you could stay in it for a long period of time. Let your head drop down in a completely relaxed way.

2 Make your breathing deep, even, and through the nostrils. Consciously direct the flow of air towards the hara. Coordinate all movements with the outbreath.

3 As you breathe out, slowly moving from the hara, shift your weight forward so that it is now focused in your palms; hold for two breaths.

4 On the next outbreath, float back to the centered position on all fours; hold for two breaths.

5 On the outbreath, shift your weight gradually forward into the left palm.

6 Roll the weight gradually into the right palm.

7 On the outbreath, return to the centered position. Repeat steps 3-7 two more times.

8 Starting from the centered position, roll your weight back so that it is focused on the knees.

9 On the outbreath, float forward to center position.

10 On the outbreath, float back into the left knee.

11 On the outbreath, roll over into the right knee.
12 On the outbreath, move diagonally forward all the way into the left palm.
13 On the outbreath, roll into the right palm.
14 On the outbreath, float diagonally back into the left knee.
15 Float forward to the centered position. Repeat steps 8-13 two more times.

During this exercise concentrate on the shifting of your weight and on how the movement originates in the hara. All movement should be done in coordination with the outbreath.

Practicing this exercise daily for several months will allow you to develop the use of your hara and give you the ability to anticipate a centered position when holding and applying pressure. Those who are already giving shiatsu should notice a dramatic change in the quality, strength, effects and results of their treatment.

Exercise 2

Crawling

As babies, all of our energy was centered and generated out from the hara. If you watch a newborn child breathe, you will see that its hara is moving in and out in a very active way. This is the reason the baby can cry so loud and strong. Although it appears as if its leg and arm motions are random, a closer look will reveal that these movements are spiralling out from the hara. At a certain point of development the baby will turn over and begin to assume the position on all fours. It then translates this native centeredness into movement through crawling. Recreating this experience is very powerful in regaining your natural centeredness, an essential quality that most of us have lost for various reasons along the way.

Once you have completed Exercise 1, begin crawling slowly around the room. Do not limit yourself. Go in all directions and shift your weight in every possible way. Follow your hara and, most of all, play and enjoy yourself.

Pressure

Pressure, in its degree and quality, is integrated within and vital to the occurrence of all physical or non-physical forms, including human life. The degree of pressure in any given phenomenon is a result of the interplay of expanding and contracting tendencies or yin and yang.

In shiatsu, developing the ability to properly and sensitively apply and create pressure is a basic key to its effectiveness and results. When an area or system of our body becomes low pressure, it does not retain the necessary life energy or ki to allow normal function and expression of the total organism. This then appears as *kyo* or *empty* energy. When we apply stimulation through touch, we create pressure at the *kyo,* inactive places and revitalize the basic life requirements.

Qualities of Energy — Kyo and Jitsu

In shiatsu, "yin" and "yang" refer more to the direction and tendency of energy. The terms *kyo* and *jitsu* apply more to the quality and degree of energy and its intensity.

Kyo   is deficient energy. It is a feeling of emptiness or being unsatisfied. *Kyo* also implies being unapparent, invisible, or hidden.

Jitsu,   on the other hand, is fullness or excess of ki energy. It appears as obvious, protruding, and overactive. *Jitsu* is easy to see; it is visible and outstanding.

Kyo is usually deep whereas *jitsu* is on the surface.

Characteristics of Kyo and Jitsu

Kyo	Jitsu
origin	compensation
empty	full
no power	resistance
hidden	projecting
wanting	result
unsatisfied	action
deep	surface

Determining *kyo* and *jitsu,* and all the variable sensations they create in the body, is the most basic assessment when interpreting the language of energy. We make this evaluation during treatment in two ways: first, through our feelings and senses, which enable us to tell if someone's energy is weak, strong, flowing, heavy, stuck, etc; second, by carefully focusing on the response we get from touching the receiver's body. Then, by connecting what we feel by our touch to what we intuitively sense, we can diagnose the condition of the person's ki energy.

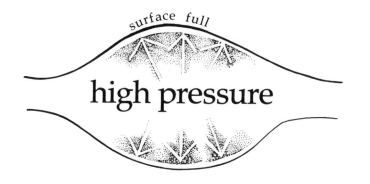

Figure 36 — Full energy of jitsu.

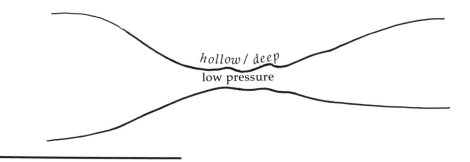

Figure 37 — Empty energy of kyo.

Pain at *kyo* points can be unpleasant and intolerable if we penetrate too quickly or with too much pressure. The body guards these areas and will quickly retract as a whole to protect its weakness. *Kyo* points will relax and open up through firm, supporting, yet gently applied pressure and through gentle stretching techniques. As these changes take place the receiver will feel a deep sense of relief. Pain at a *jitsu* area is more bearable and superficial. The person will usually only experience this reaction at the point where pressure is applied. A *kyo* condition first develops on the level of the body's energy system and can then further cause a deficiency in body movement, organ, or system activity. This *kyo* condition creates the need for some other function to become more active, full, or *jitsu*, a resulting action of the innate compensating mechanism of all phenomena in nature. With *jitsu*, an emphasis of energy develops in one or several meridians and their related body areas in order to harmonize the organism as a whole. This generally appears as being overly strong and seems, on the surface, to be the source of the receiver's problem. However the need for this excess action is continually generated deep inside by *kyo*. Acute or less serious imbalance of *kyo* and *jitsu* tend only to appear in the meridians and in the person's overall energetic quality. These conditions of a lesser degree can, however, mildly affect the function of organs and produce various symptoms.

In diagnosis we will often find that the particular meridians and related body areas that are affected by acute imbalance will change from treatment to treatment. Long-term or chronic imbalances cause more serious dysfunction of the organs and body systems with prolonged, uncomfortable symptoms. Along with greater distortion of the meridians, the body will develop pronounced postural misalignments. These chronic imbalances will tend to remain within the same meridians and body areas, producing the same symptoms again and again.

One of the mistakes many inexperienced practitioners make is to focus on the *jitsu* distortions of the body and its energy system rather than seek to discover the causal, underlying *kyo*. Again this is because *jitsu* places are apparent while *kyo* is hiding.

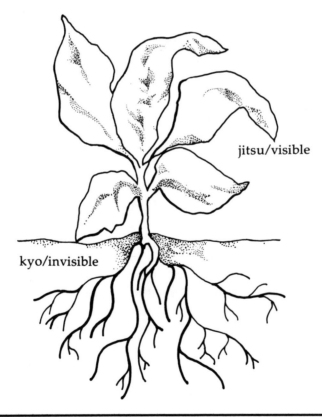

Figure 38 — A kyo/jitsu imbalance is like a weed growing in the garden. If we pull out only the leaves, the roots grow deeper.

Working on a *jitsu* place brings more energy and attention to an area that already has an excess. In the case of a weak, chronically ill person, it can make their condition worse. Using the properly applied technique of the Basic Frame Outline presented in the next section, we can encourage the receiver to relax and open up the flow of their energy. Gradually they will allow us to see their weakness as the *kyo* comes out to the surface. As we practice and become more sensitive, we will be able to identify these weaknesses more quickly, and in an unobtrusive way. We can then strengthen the *kyo* area, meridian or point which will then allow the *jitsu* to relax and dissolve.

The *kyo/jitsu* that appears in the body as a result of energy imbalances will also permeate all other levels of expression such as emotions, intellect, psychology, activity, preferences and view of life.

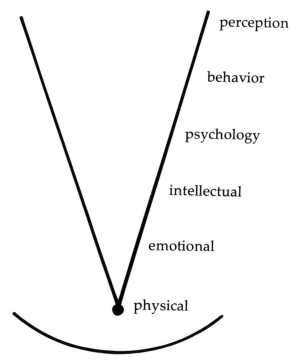

Energy Systems

Figure 39 —

Examples of Kyo and Jitsu

The following are a few examples of the many ways that *kyo* and *jitsu* can appear and be expressed.

Kyo-jitsu relationship	Related symptoms, conditions and life expressions
Kidney meridian: *jitsu* Large Intestine meridian: *kyo*	Loose stools, frequent urination, tightness in lower back of legs, dark hue around the face, lack of expression.
Spleen meridian: *jitsu* Heart meridian: *kyo*	Person feels wanting and unfulfilled in terms of being loved; this creates empty heart energy. To compensate they overeat from frustration. Spleen becomes *jitsu*.
Gallbladder meridian: *jitsu* Lung meridian: *kyo*	Person lacks sociability. They have a fear of being rejected. This attitude is a result of *kyo* in the lungs and related body areas. (See Diagnosis) To compensate, gallbladder becomes *jitsu*, creating a tight clenched jaw, incomplete communications, and irregular elimination. This person will become over-extended in work and overlook relaxation time.
Left side of body: *jitsu* Right side of body: *kyo*	Left side appears larger and moves more. There is a tendency to strain and injure the left side from overuse. This person tends to be very physical and aggressive and lacks gentleness and patience. They have a tendency to develop a weak bond and poor relations with their mother and other female authority figures.
Exterior: *jitsu* Interior: *kyo*	This is a very general example of how the body appearance expresses long-term psychological imbalance. This person creates a hard, muscular, external appearance and a tough expression. Internally they experience great fear of being loved and letting others know they crave attention and acceptance. Physically they can experience digestive problems and circulatory disorders. The original cause is the intake of animal food and sugar, and stems psychologically from the rejection of parents.

To have this judgement of *kyo* and *jitsu* we need to develop our sense of energy and not to rely on our sense of the physical alone. Physical qualities such as hard, soft, tight, etc., are an expression of various conditions of energy; two very similar physical qualities can have opposite energetic causes. To use physical information as the sole basis of diagnosis can therefore be misleading and inaccurate. As an example we can use the sensations of squeezing a rubber hose. If water is running through without obstruction, the hose feels full and at the same time has give. When we push the hose in, there is the power and resilience to push back. This is similar to a balanced feeling when applying pressure to a healthy person's body. If we run water through the hose and crimp the end so that the water becomes trapped inside, the hose will feel hard to the touch and the built-up pressure will give us a feeling of fullness. This resembles the feeling of *jitsu*. If the hose is empty and lying outside in freezing weather, it will still feel hard on the outside. However our senses can tell us that the inside is empty. This is similar to a place on the body that has become chronically *kyo* and has built up a lot of surface protection.

Recognizing *kyo* and *jitsu* takes time, patience, and the experience of many treatments. We must first become sensitive simply to the variations and qualities of energy we feel under our hands. In time, and with plenty of practice, you will know what the condition of energy is. In our style of shiatsu we always seek to find the *kyo* meridian, body area or point. This is the origin of the imbalance. When strengthened, it will allow the tense, *jitsu* place to relax.

The following exercises progressively develop our sensitivity to and interpretation of energetic qualities:

Exercise 1
Feeling seven levels of energy in each point or tsubo.

Practice the following exercises on yourself and then on someone else. They develop the ability to distinguish depth and layers of energy within each tsubo.

1. Touch a point at the top of your thigh, right at the surface.
2. As you breathe out, slowly sink into the tsubo, counting seven different levels.
3. Tune carefully into the different sensations and qualities of the seven levels.
4. By the seventh level, you should have the sensation of being at the bottom of the tsubo.
5. Hold at the bottom of the tsubo and wait.
6. Release gently; move to another area and start again.
7. Pick up a line from the first point at the top of the thigh down to the ankle and do each point along this line carefully.

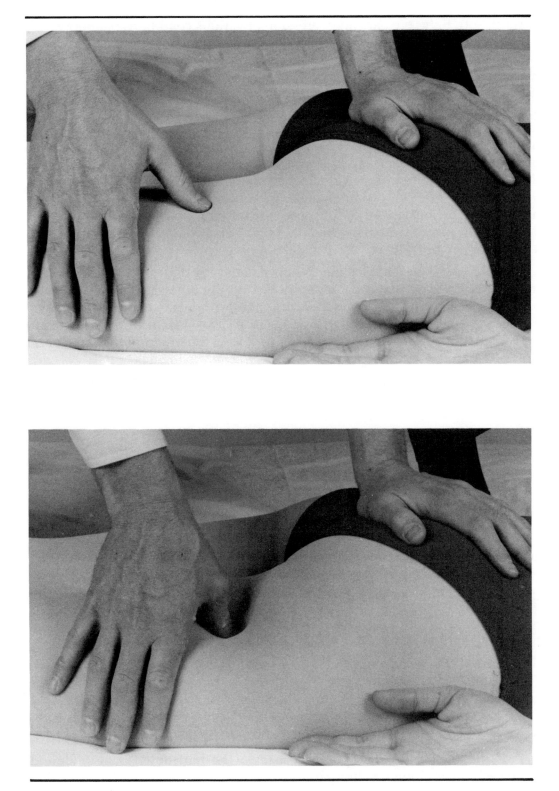

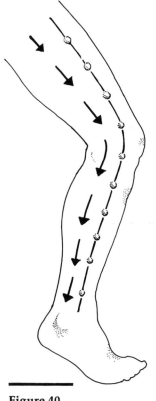

Figure 40 —

It may be helpful to keep your eyes closed. This will make your sense of touch sharper and prevent visual distractions. Practice this exercise on the head, arm, hand, foot, etc. It will enable you to begin sensing the character of tsubos and their energy in different places of the body.

Repeat these exercises on a partner.

——————— Exercise 2 ———————

Feeling the shift from orthosympathetic to parasympathetic: separated to unified.

In many shiatsu books it is suggested that the practitioner hold each point for 3-7 seconds while applying about 10 lbs. of pressure. This is a very mechanical guideline. In practice, our approach must be flexible. Every person and every tsubo has a different quality, character, and requirement, making it essential that we feel and become sensitive to what is happening under our hands.

It is important to patiently hold each tsubo when you reach its bottom or as far as it will allow you to penetrate. At this place you will feel a separation between your hand or thumb, and the receiver's body. As you hold, focusing from hara, you will feel this separation melt away. This is followed by the feeling that you and the receiver are 'one' at the place of contact.

1. Practice sinking in carefully and hold each point along a chosen line on a body area, similar to the preceding exercise.

2. When the separation dissolves the point is energetically active and in connection with the body energy system which ultimately functions as a whole. Often it takes time to feel this shift in sensation. A longer time shows resistance at a more surface level, protecting weakness deeper in the point. This is a weakness created by a *kyo* or energy-deficient condition. If you hold in a very supportive way, then this protective resistance eventually gives way. At this point energy is coming through to the area where you are applying pressure.

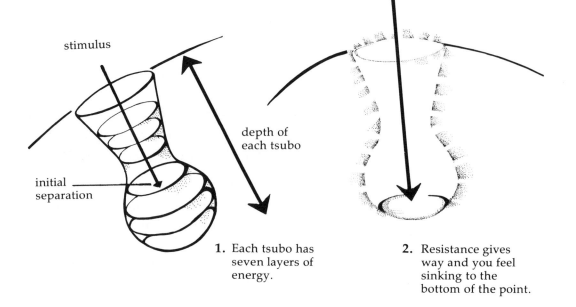

stimulus

depth of each tsubo

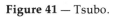

initial separation

1. Each tsubo has seven layers of energy.

2. Resistance gives way and you feel sinking to the bottom of the point.

Figure 41 — Tsubo.

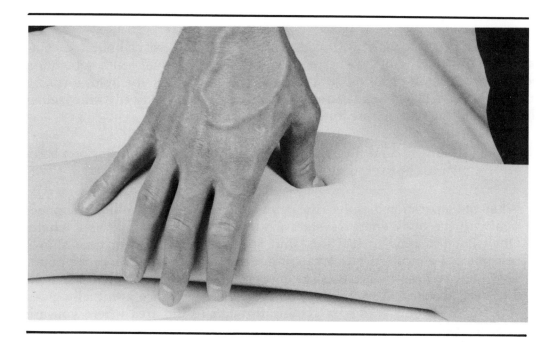

3. The amount of holding time for each point is until the feeling of separation dissolves; this will vary from immediate opening to about 45 seconds. If it takes any longer then go on to another place and continue your treatment. Come back later to the tsubo and try again. With some points you may also get the feeling of only partial opening. This also requires that you return to the point later on in the treatment session.

4. When you first sink into most points you will feel that the receiver is only receiving the stimulus locally. This is the orthosympathetic-related mechanism processing the intent behind the stimulus and keeping it outside of the body.

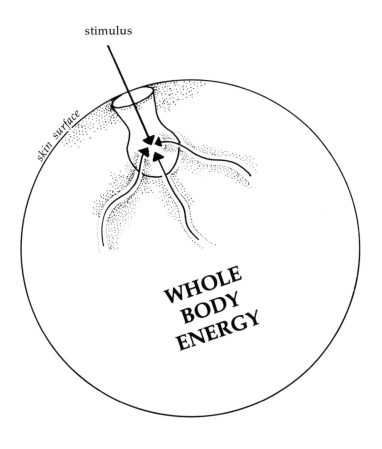

Figure 42 — Local reception — the receiver feels stimulus only at the local point of contact. The receiver is conscious of the stimulus. The giver experiences separation.

As you hold patiently, the stimulus will begin to filter or wave out and you will sense that it is now being received by the body as a whole unit. This sensation arises from the increased activity of the parasympathetic senses.

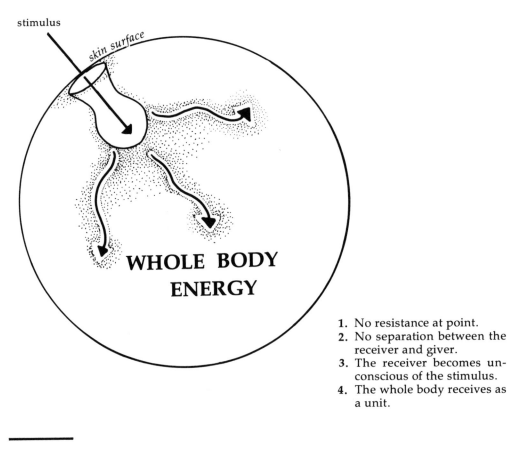

1. No resistance at point.
2. No separation between the receiver and giver.
3. The receiver becomes unconscious of the stimulus.
4. The whole body receives as a unit.

Figure 43 —

5. When the separation dissolves you will feel yourself sink into the bottom of the point. This is actually a very minute distance (not to scale on the drawing) so you must pay careful attention to the sensation under your hands.

───────────────────── **Exercise 3** ─────────────────────
Using two hands

In shiatsu we use both hands together as often as possible. One hand is generally stationary; we call this the *support* hand. The other hand is the active or *moving* hand. The moving hand usually goes out from the support hand, stimulating and opening tsubos. The support hand, being stationary, adapts itself to the body and gives a constant underlying charge to the parasympathetic system. This gives the receiver more confidence and ability in opening up to the action of the moving hand. Because it continues to trigger the body-adapting mechanism, the support hand allows the receiver to maintain a state of relaxation and realize all of the related benefits.

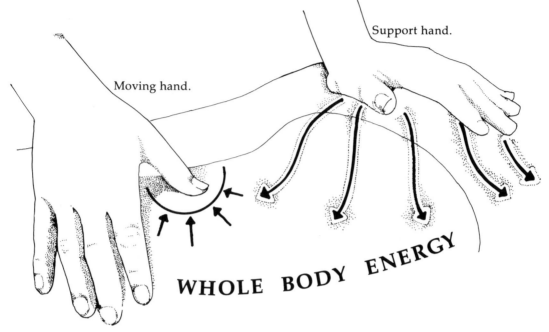

Figure 44 — Support Hand: adapts and becomes connected with body sense of wholeness via energy system. Moving Hand: contacts point and waits for adaptation to occur.

The support hand adapts and becomes connected with body sense of wholeness via energy system.

The moving hand contacts points and waits for adaptation to occur.

When the support hand is patiently holding and applying steady even pressure, the giver experiences the feeling of oneness with the receiver in that hand. Meanwhile the moving hand is going through the separation-to-unification process, as discussed in Exercise 2.

When the moving hand is unified at each point, the practitioner feels oneness at this point and with the receiver's whole body. He also feels as if his two hands become as one. There is a distinct current of energy running between the two hands and the receiver experiences the two contact places of the practitioner's hands as if it were one large surface of contact. Once you can continuously create this sensation for yourself and the receiver, the effect of your treatment will become much stronger.

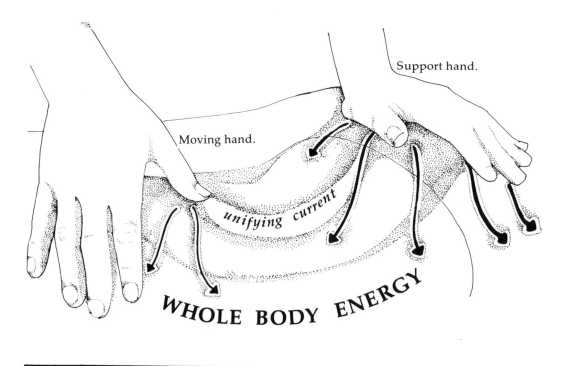

Figure 45 — Resistance gives way, two hands unite and current runs between the hands.

In treatment this technique usually affects the receiver in the following way: At first you will feel a small section of the body relax where you are working; then a larger area will give way; finally the entire body will shift. This is a turning point in the treatment and means that the whole energy system is open and flowing. At this point you can make many fine adjustments. You must stay constantly focused on the treatment and keep your attention in your hara to sense the receiver's energetic responses while you are working. When this becomes an automatic habit, then the appropriate technique and how to proceed in the treatment will always present itself with no effort.

It is necessary to keep your attention on both hands and hara at the same time. Practice this technique in the following ways:

1. Place the support hand on the sacrum.

2. Draw three imaginary lines down the back of the leg.

3. Give pressure down each line.

4. Hold each point until separation dissolves and both your hands are connected by a current of energy.

Also practice with the support hand on the shoulder and the active hand giving shiatsu along three lines on the arm.

Practice with the support hand at the base of the neck and the active hand going down a line along the back.

It is helpful to wear a blindfold while practicing in order to exclude visual distractions.

Exercises 1, 2, and 3 should be practiced separately for one to two weeks at a time. Begin with Exercise 1 and progress to Exercise 3. Developing and executing these skills of technique, concentration and sensitivity in the proper way will make your shiatsu strong, with a deep penetration and long-lasting results. Take your time and master each one separately. When confident that you are feeling these sensations of energy and changing response, begin using your knee, elbow, and forearm in place of the moving hand. These parts of the body create a more penetrating, powerful pressure, with a wider base of coverage, so be very cautious and sensitive when beginning to use them.

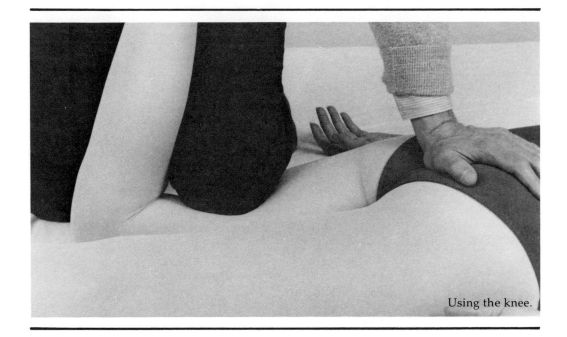

Using the knee.

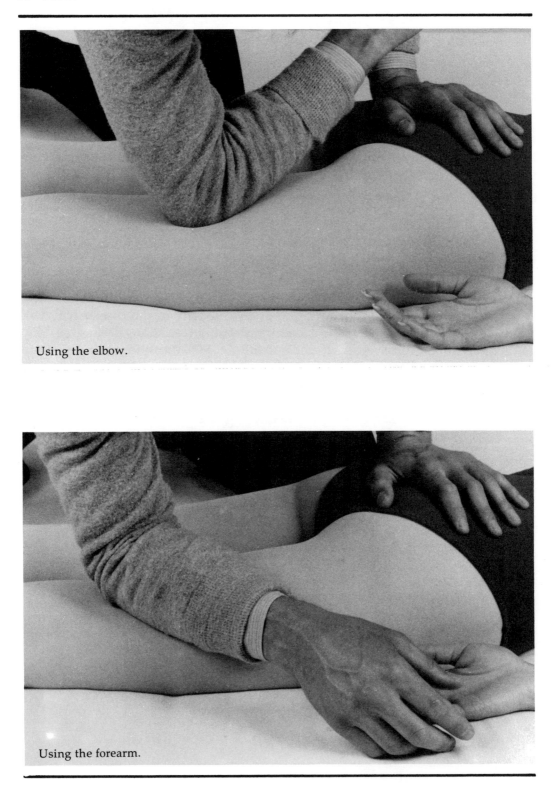

Using the elbow.

Using the forearm.

General Exercises

The following exercises are to develop the awareness of how energy manifests with different characteristics in the world around us. If we become conscious of the various elements involved in these exercises as a representation of energetic interplay, we can gain some interesting insights into the order and universal involvements of energy. These exercises will help us see that what we experience in shiatsu is directly related to all other experiences in work and play. Developing this sense of energetic interplay allows shiatsu to enhance our daily experiences and vice versa.

Exercise 1

1. Gather 5 different types of balls.
2. Close your eyes, pick up each ball separately and squeeze it.
3. Bounce each one up and down in your hand.
4. Feel the difference in resilience, texture, weight (pull of gravity), etc.
5. Repeat steps 2-4 with a ball in each hand.

Exercise 2

1. Choose 5 or 6 different textured surfaces.
2. With your eyes closed, rub each one.
3. Mentally describe the different qualities and characteristics of each surface. Examples: rough, smooth, fuzzy, harsh, bristled.

Exercise 3

1. Drive three or four different automobiles in succession.
2. Distinguish the difference in pressure and resilience in the brake pedal of each vehicle.
3. Experience the different level of power from the drive of each engine.
4. Feel the different levels of play and response in the individual steering devices.

Notice that, when driving, the individual operations are performed with the same exchange of body movement and mechanical change, yet, from vehicle to vehicle, they require different amounts of pressure, strength, and various speeds of application in order to achieve the desired results.

The Basic Frame Outline

The course at our shiatsu center in Bucks County, Pennsylvania, requires that students,whether or not they have any previous experience, attend a weekend intensive. Here they are presented with the fundamentals of shiatsu philosophy, similar to what you have read so far, and what we call the Basic Frame Outline.

The purpose of the Basic Frame Outline is to develop a large context in which to see and treat people. It allows the student to incorporate all further studies including standard shiatsu technique, their own personal innovations, swedish massage work, body integration methods, structural alignment technique, and energy healing processes. We stress that they develop their shiatsu practice and personal studies within this broad outline.

The outline encourages us to look at the people to whom we give shiatsu in the most wholistic way. We begin by seeing them as a total condition of ki energy which is functioning as a whole unit. Once we are able to perceive this largest, most simple view, the details, such as seeing the location of meridians, points, and structural relationships, fall easily into place. On the other hand, if we become initially concerned with specifics, we may lose track of, or never see the total picture.

Our human constitution is made up of twelve major meridians plus two special meridians. Then there are also supplementary energy flows, internal and external passages, and their connecting systems. Together this adds up to sixty-four energy passageways. There are 360 major acupuncture points, the six major organic systems, the structural framework of bones and muscles, and several detailed systems of diagnosis. You can see from this that details can easily become a hopeless maze if we begin from a tunnel vision perspective. I have seen many students fall into the trap of trying to memorize and use all of this information while never being able to produce a simple and fluent shiatsu treatment.

When we start within a unifying context and continuously practice, the details arrange themselves within it. We begin to naturally see the meridians, points, energy distortions, and structural misalignments. Eventually the emotional, psychological and life experience of the person receiving shiatsu presents itself to us as if we were viewing a motion picture.

Our ongoing program at the center hones in on the specifics of developing a full, well-rounded practice. Students study technique, diagnosis, and personal development which incorporates specific dietary awareness for healing. This is all taught within the Basic Frame orientation. In the final stages of study the students are encouraged to develop spontaneity and to finally become free of the frame structure.

Although the Basic Frame Outline is simple it provides a very powerful, full body shiatsu. When applied properly, it will effect a very strong treatment. Please go slowly in learning and practicing. Speed is not important. Each time we learn something new, we not only need to know it conceptually, we need to experience it practically in order to understand and make it valuable. Be concerned mostly with the quality of your work and think as little as possible about degrees, certifications, or reimbursements for your time. When there is quality in your work, these smaller considerations naturally take care of themselves.

General Guidelines For Giving Shiatsu

The following guidelines are important to understand prior to giving shiatsu. They create a condition or mind-set for the practitioner that encourages an optimum environment in which to produce the maximum results.

1. Empty Stomach

It is best to be empty inside when giving shiatsu. This makes the nervous system highly charged and you become more sensitive to vibrations. On the other hand, if the stomach is full, energy is diverted to the digestive vessels and your sensitivity is reduced. You should leave about two and a half hours between eating and giving treatment. However, if you feel hungry or weak, it is fine to take a very light meal of high quality grain/vegetable food.

2. Empty Mind

'Empty mind' is another classic attitude of ancient, spiritually oriented peoples. It means that we approach each situation and the multiple factors involved as unique. We must drop all our pretentions and concepts so that we can receive the real picture in any given moment. This holds true when giving treatment in that if our minds are full of what meridian is imbalanced, what points need stimulation, or what the receiver's problem is related to, we can be blocked from seeing the condition that is really there. If our mind is still and we allow the hara to guide us, we will know what needs to be done and how to do it.

To give strong shiatsu we need three things:
- A simple, broad context
- To work from hara
- An empty mind

3. Never use force — support only.

When we try to force things in life it creates the opposite of what we seek to achieve. For instance, if you coerce someone into eating healthy foods they will eventually go to junk food. If you try to force someone onto a spiritual path they will become more materialistic than before. The unconscious body works by the same mechanism. If we force it in a direction that it does not want to go in, with the intention of stimulating energy or of making it more flexible, we actually produce more tension and constriction.

The body opens up and energy flows when a person becomes relaxed. In order to do this we must make them feel supported at all levels of our interchange. In treatment, always position or move the body in a way which allows it to relax and be comfortable. Pressure, stretching or rotating actions should be applied in a gradual, gentle, and firm way. *Allow the body to adapt to each procedure according to its own capacity* and not to a preconceived idea that you have of how flexible or resilient it should be.

The receiver has generally come for shiatsu because they sense something is imbalanced or stuck in their body, mind and life. Knowing this, it is not necessary to immediately bring attention to the weakness or imbalances that you see. This approach will put the person on guard, making them protective and closed, along with creating difficulty for them in opening up, relaxing, trusting, and letting go. These conditions, although they may be unconscious, then carry over into and inhibit the treatment.

It is best to initially find some common ground of communication with which the receiver feels comfortable. Then, as in all levels of interchange, the person will begin to open up and reveal their weaknesses and problems to you. Communicating on a common ground establishes trust and confidence by allowing the receiver to come forward and open up at their own pace instead of being pried open by pointed, leading questions. Once their guard is down they will tend to progressively relax and open throughout the treatment.

4. Continuity

The word continuity means 'con': with, and 'tinuity': unity. The movement in shiatsu should flow from one stage to the next, creating the treatment as a whole. Continuity in the application of our technique gives the receiver a sense of trust and unification with the practitioner. It allows them to confidently open up and relax. If the practitioner jumps around from one technique to another or from one body area or position to another, the receiver becomes suspicious of their ability. Fragmentation in treatment makes separation and closes off the exchange of energy between the giver and receiver. For this reason, I recommend that the student practice each step of the Basic Frame Outline technique in the given order until it becomes one whole, flowing motion.

5. Use Two Hands

Develop a 'two hand consciousness' and apply it as often as possible. This means our attention is directed to the response being felt by each hand at the same time. (See Exercise 3, page 64.) This approach will effect a deep unification of the receiver's energy systems.

6. Natural Environment and Clothing

Natural cotton clothing allows a smooth interchange of energy between the practitioner and client. Documented research now shows that unnatural fabrics decrease the capacity of our biological functions, particularly those related to the nervous system. Using natural materials in the environment where you are giving shiatsu encourages maximum movement of energy. Unnatural lighting and artificial articles, along with electrically operated devices, create an environment of more (+) positively charged ions therefore interrrupting, blocking, or stagnating the normal current of energy flow.

7. Sincere Desire and Clear Intention

This is the most important point of all. If our desire and intention are clear we need very little technical training in order to develop our practice.

Intention is the way in which we internally direct our ki energy, and desire is what we seek to create. Always remember that the purpose in giving shiatsu is the benefit of the receiver. Our benefit and reward is automatically built in to the opportunity to serve and give. We should always seek to make the people we work with feel better, lighter and more relaxed by helping them create a condition of balance.

When I studied shiatsu many fellow students were able to perform beautiful technique with graceful movement; however, the treatment was weak in effect and unsatisfying to the receiver. This was because they had focused so much attention on techique and its correctness, along with taking personal pride in the execution. Unfortunately they overlooked or lost track of the purpose of giving shiatsu. On the other hand I have observed interactions where a person was feeling tired, stiff, or depressed and a friend spontaneously began to give them pressure, stretching or kneading stimulation. Even though they had no previous training or had at best observed someone else giving shiatsu, the effect was very strong and the receiver felt much better. These opposite results were due to the nature of the intention and desire. Please examine this closely when giving shiatsu; it will determine what you bring forth.

Our goal is to strike empathy and compassion for the receiver and all that they feel and experience. Our touch and support is similar to the comfort we give a friend who is feeling low. Just by putting our arm around their shoulder they automatically feel better and lighten up. This support also resembles the touch a mother gives a crying baby. Just through rocking and holding, the child is soothed and relaxed.

If we give this feeling in shiatsu, the results will be very strong and powerful. We should always strive to make this our basic orientation in treatment as well as in our day-to-day life.

Basic Frame Outline

Technique and Practice

Basic Frame Outline — Technique and Practice

The first impression we give the recipient sets the tone for our treatment. If we make the person feel uncomfortable, distrustful or not confident through our initial touch, this will carry through for the whole treatment. Before we begin we should center ourselves by bringing our focus to hara, clearing our mind, relaxing, and reviewing our intentions.

Centering

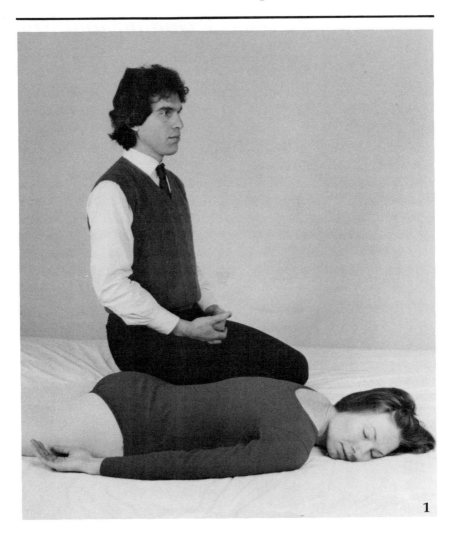

1 Sit in *seiza* or natural sitting position. Make sure your spine is straight.

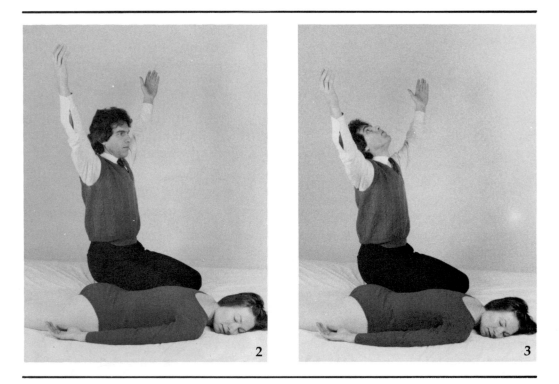

2 As you breathe out, let the hands float up above the head; keep your elbows straight.

3 On the next outbreath, let the head float back so that you are looking up at your hands.

4 Breathing out, let the head float back to the erect position.

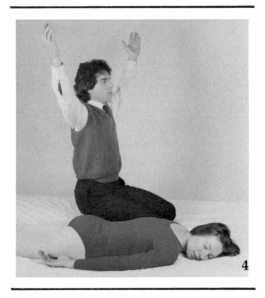

5 As you breathe out, let the hands slowly float down and rest them for a few seconds in your lap. Breathe naturally, in a relaxed way. These movements straighten your spine and allow a full charge of energy to flow through the body's main energy channel.

6 Next, rub the hands together briskly until they become very warm. The heat shows that energy is now circulating out to the periphery of your body.

A With the right hand make a tight fist around the pinky of the left hand and rotate strongly.

B Rotate each finger. Repeat on the right hand.

C Again briskly rub the hands together.

6

D Hold the palms 12 inches apart. If the mind is quiet and you are focused in the hara, you will feel a current of ki energy moving between the hands. This feels like an invisible cushion.

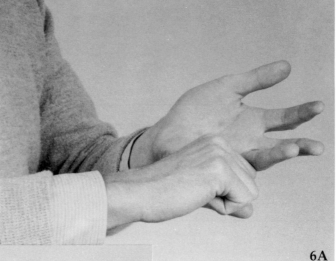

6A

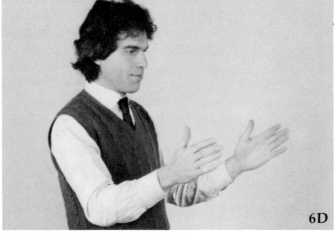

6D

7 Breathe deeply and evenly through the nostrils for about 30 seconds.

The Basic Frame Outline • 79

Order of Treatment

The Basic Frame Outline will go through the body in the following order:

1. Back
2. Legs and Feet
3. Arms and Hands
4. Shoulders and Neck
5. Head and Face

- Begin working on the LEFT side of the body and work round to the RIGHT side.

- For information on the practitioner's position, please pay close attention to the photographs.

The Back

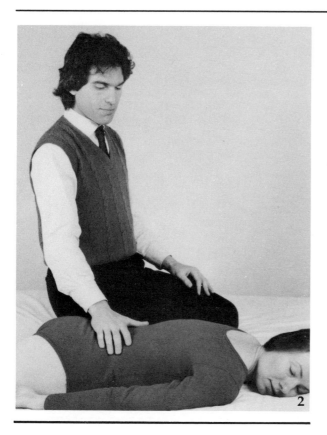

1 Sit in seiza, to the left of the receiver.
While sitting in a very relaxed way, try to imagine what it would be like to be in the receiver's body and to have their mind. Feel them as a whole unit of ki energy.

2 Gently and firmly lay your right hand on the small of the receiver's back. Again assess their overall energy.

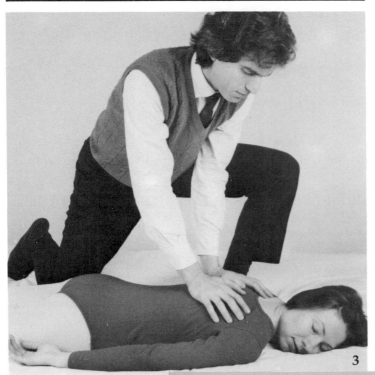

3 Place both palms on either side of the spine on the upper back. Using your weight, sink in, giving pressure as you both breathe out. Hold for a few seconds at the end of each outbreath.

Continue down the back until you reach the lower back; repeat three times. (See Diagnosis, Part 7).

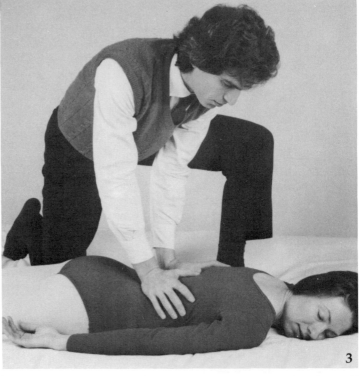

4 Make your right hand like a knife. (*knife hand*)
With your left hand placed on the receiver's tailbone (sacrum), make a penetrating, saw-like motion with the fingertips of the right hand all the way down the back, alongside the spine. Do this on each side of the spine three times.

Note: This is a sawing, not a rubbing motion. It can penetrate deeply as long as the receiver does not tense their body.

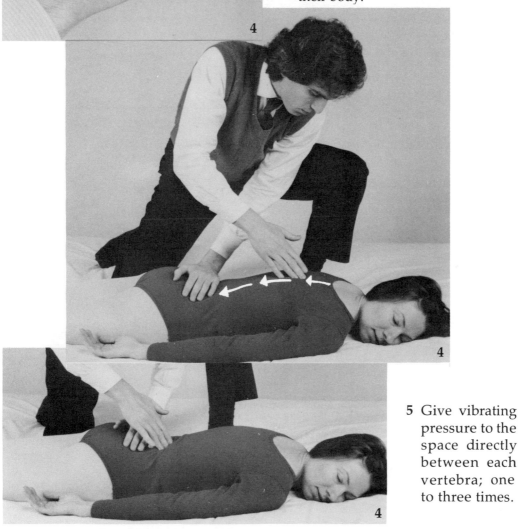

5 Give vibrating pressure to the space directly between each vertebra; one to three times.

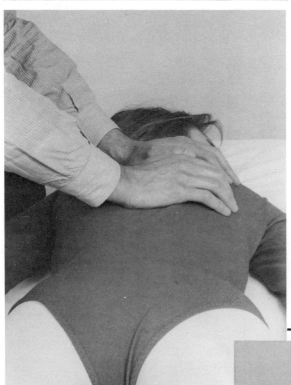

6 Rocking:
A Place the heel of the hands in the space between the scapula and spine on the side closest to you.

B Begin to rock the receiver back and forth so that their entire body moves in a wave-like motion. The heels of your hands are rolling over the band-like *sacro-spinalis* muscles.

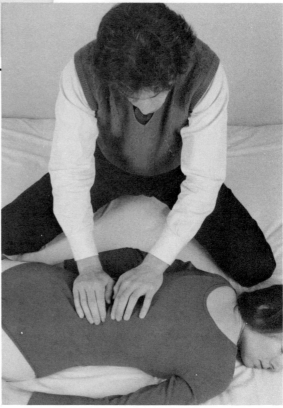

C As you continue to rock, move the right hand down the back and follow with the left hand, alternately moving the hands until you come to the lower back.

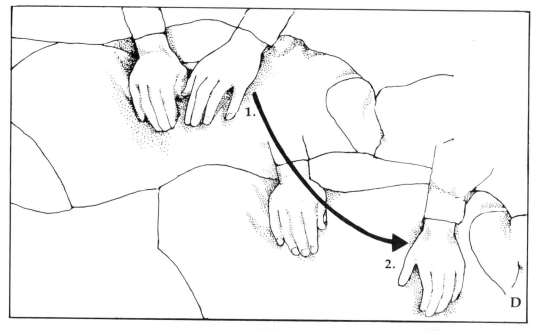

D When you reach the small of the back, continue to rock with the right hand and reach up to the top of the receiver's right side with the left hand. Follow with the right hand.

　(2) Continue working down the back alternating hands. Repeat the whole technique three times.

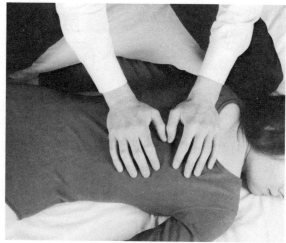

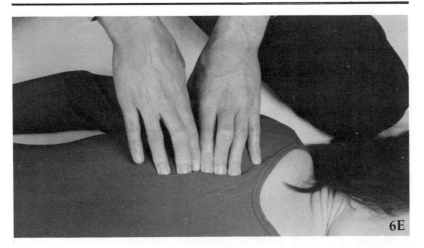

E Using the fingertips instead of the heels of the hands, repeat steps A-D.

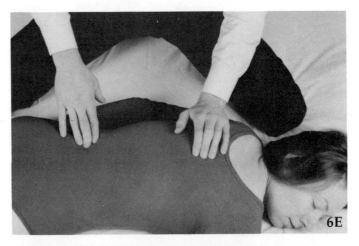

F Allow the receiver's body to come to rest slowly. Hold your right hand on their lower back, until you feel warmth pass between their back and your hand.

Remove your hand slowly. If you are focused, you will sense that the receiver feels as though they are still rocking and as if your hand is still on their body. This type of penetration begins to trigger the body's relaxation mechanisms, allowing energy to begin flowing.

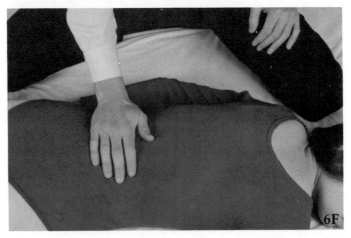

7 **The Bladder Meridian:** The bladder meridian is the only meridian we will be concerned with in the Basic Frame Outline. Its energy charges the autonomic nervous system and it connects directly to the other eleven major meridians. The bladder meridian splits into two branches along either side of the spine. These are called Bladder 1 and Bladder 2 respectively.

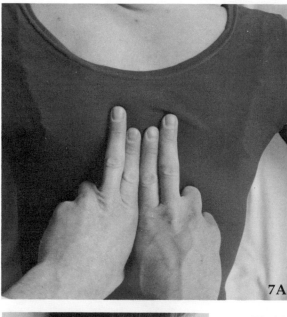

7A

A To find Bladder 1 measure out two fingers' width from the very center of the spine.

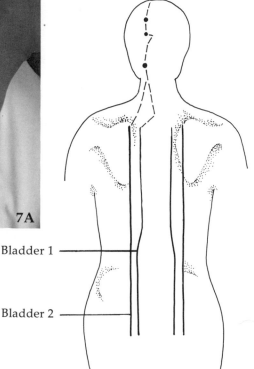

Bladder 1

Bladder 2

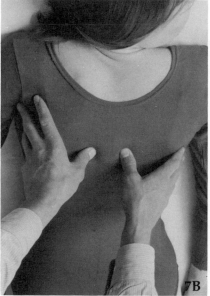

7B

B Starting at the top of the back, give pressure to each tsubo* down the back. Hold pressure until you feel the separation-unification shift. Repeat three times.

C To find Bladder 2 measure four fingers width out from the center of the spine.

(1) Give pressure on each tsubo from the top of the back to the bottom.

*Tsubos are about 1" apart; however don't worry about exact location. Eventually, with practice, your thumbs will go to the right place. Creating good quality pressure, along with proper time of holding, is more the initial concern.

Repeat up to three times. Both giver and receiver breathe out as the thumb sinks into each tsubo. While holding, they both breathe according to their natural rhythm.

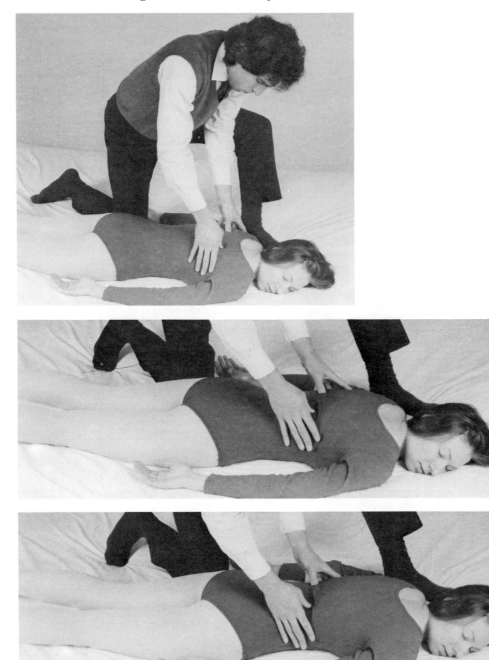

8 The Scapula (Shoulder Blade)

Move up to the shoulders. Gently bounce the shoulders together and then alternately. (Pages 87, 88, 89). This helps us gauge the receiver's range of motion.

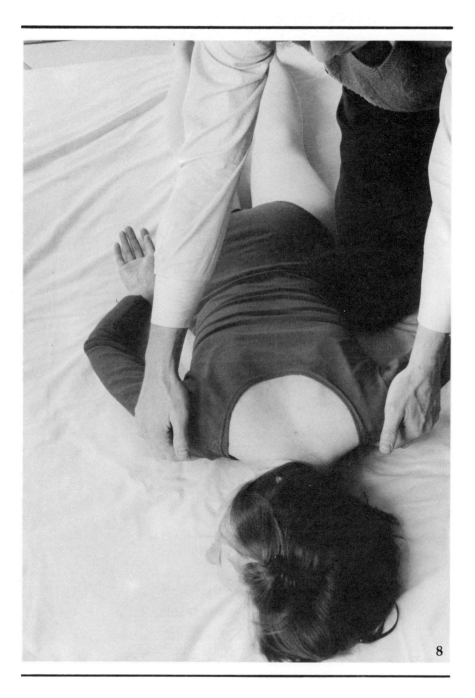

8

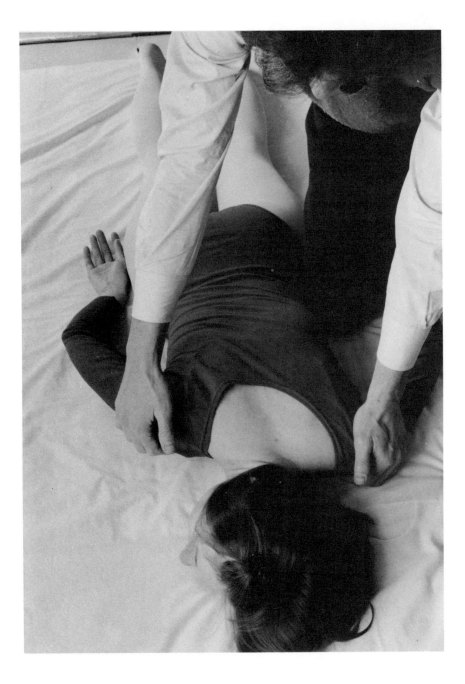

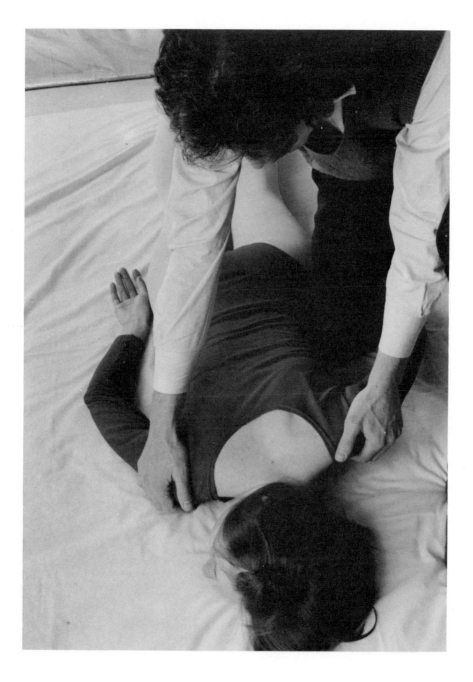

A Bend the arm around the back. Be considerate of receiver's bending capacity.

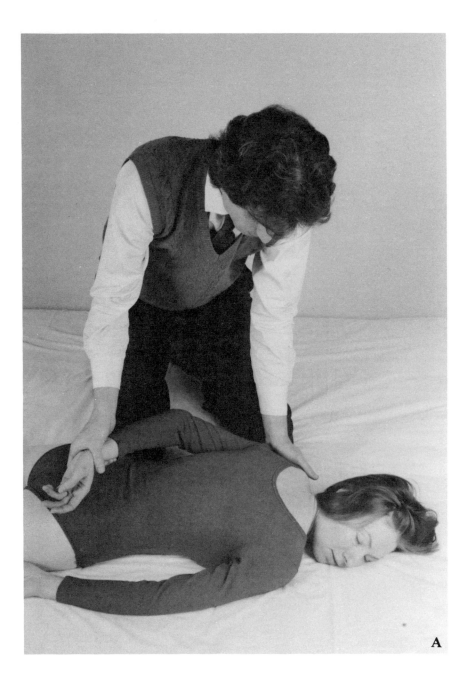

B Hold the arm in place with the leg closest to their body.

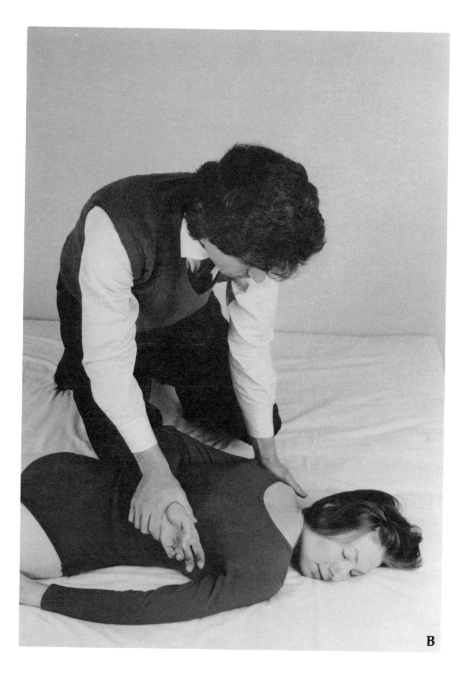

C Raise the shoulder with your outside hand.

D Gently bounce the shoulder, observing the movement of the scapula (shoulder blade).

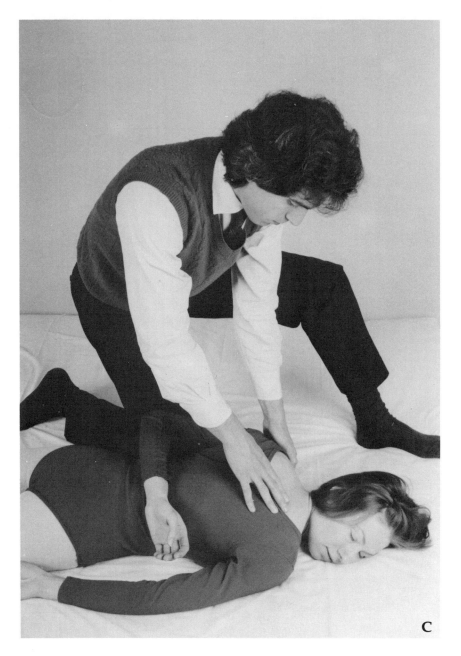

C

E Place the thumb at the top of the vertebral border of the scapula.

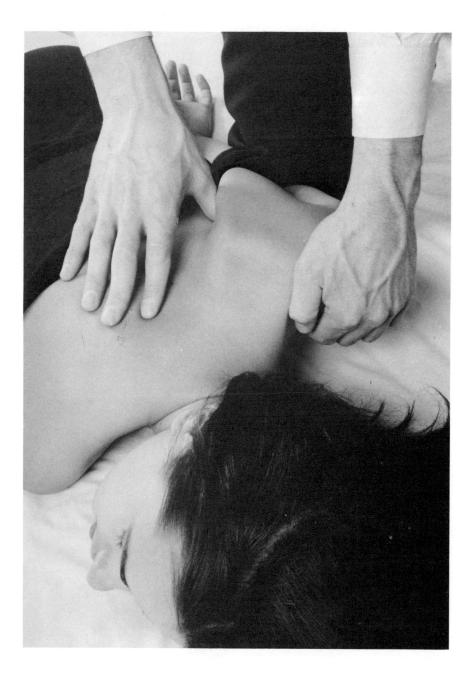

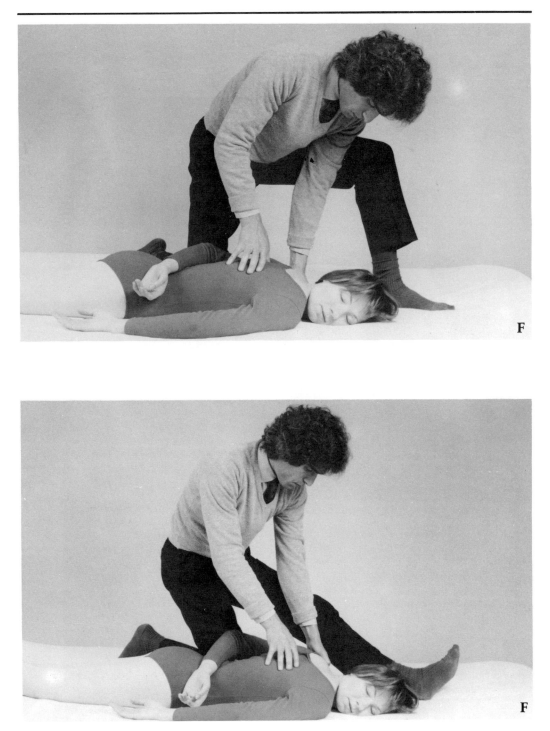

F   Shift your weight back from the hara and, as the scapula rises, allow your thumb to sink in and under.

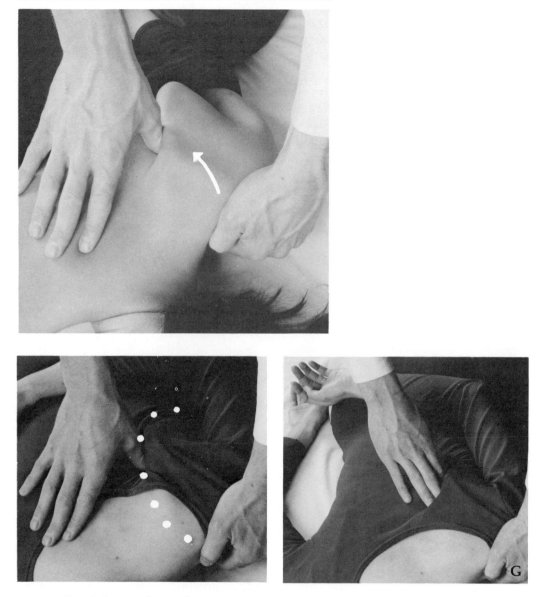

Do all of the tsubos along
the border, allowing proper
holding time.

G If the shoulder area appears to be stuck, start this technique by first
actively moving the scapula up and down, thrusting a 'knife hand' under
the scapula. Once you sense that energy is moving use holding pressure
all along the border, as described in step F.

9 Move so that you are sitting at the receiver's head.

    A Place the heels of your hands at the upper edges of the shoulder blades.

    B Rock the whole body by directing your focus of ki towards and out through their feet.

    C Rock both shoulders together and then alternately.

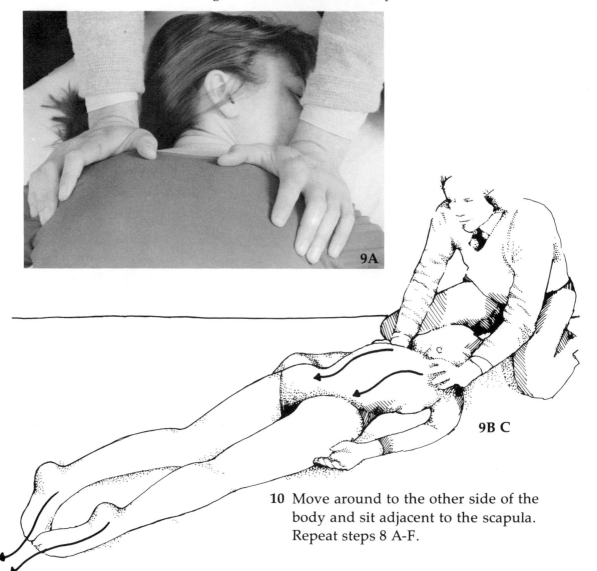

9A

9B C

10 Move around to the other side of the body and sit adjacent to the scapula. Repeat steps 8 A-F.

11 The Sacrum

The *sacrum* is the plate-like bone at the base of the spine. It has five notches on each descending border called *foramen*. To locate the foramen notches find the two ball-like protrusions where the hip joins the sacrum. The foramen lie directly to the inside of and just below these protrusions.

A Give pressure in each notch on both sides using the thumbs; repeat one to three times.

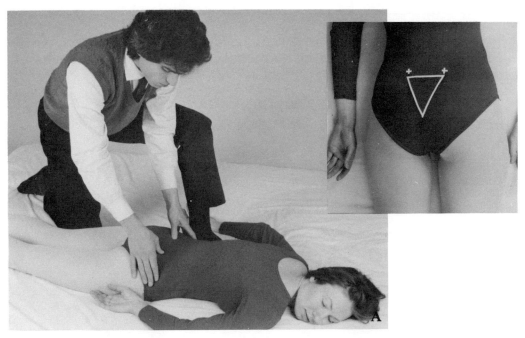

B Overlap the hands and hold them over the sacrum. On the outbreath, give pressure.

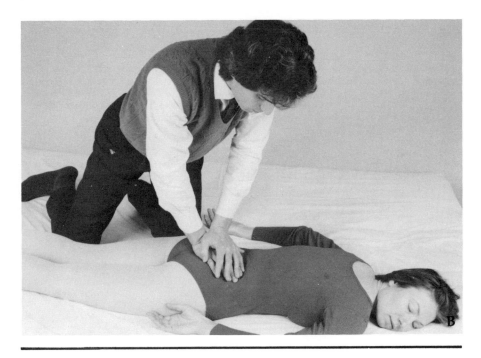

Legs and Feet

1 Begin by using a simultaneous squeezing, kneading, rolling motion from the top of the thigh to the ankle. This encourages energy to begin moving towards the lower sphere of the body.

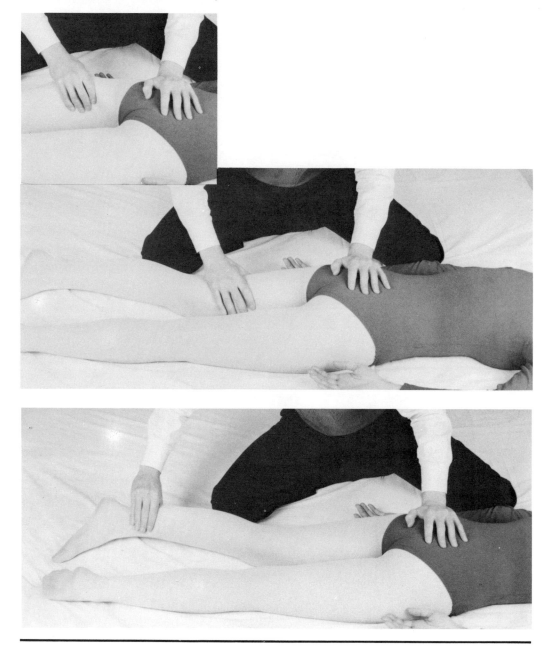

2 Place the hand which is nearer to the receiver's head over the sacrum. This remains stationary and becomes the support hand.

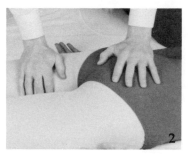

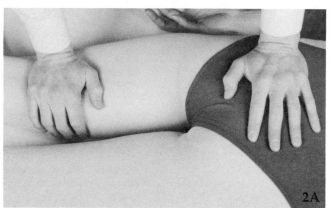

A Using the hand which is closer to the feet, give holding pressure with the palm down the center of the thigh and calf.

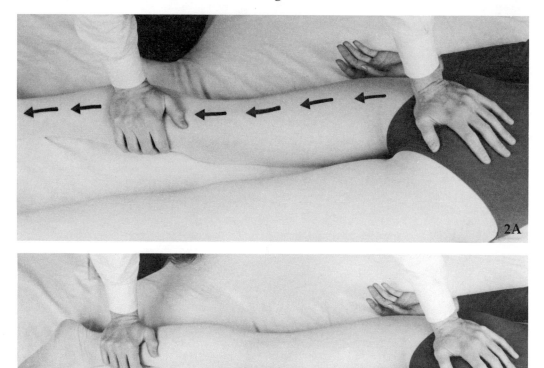

B Repeat step A using your thumb.

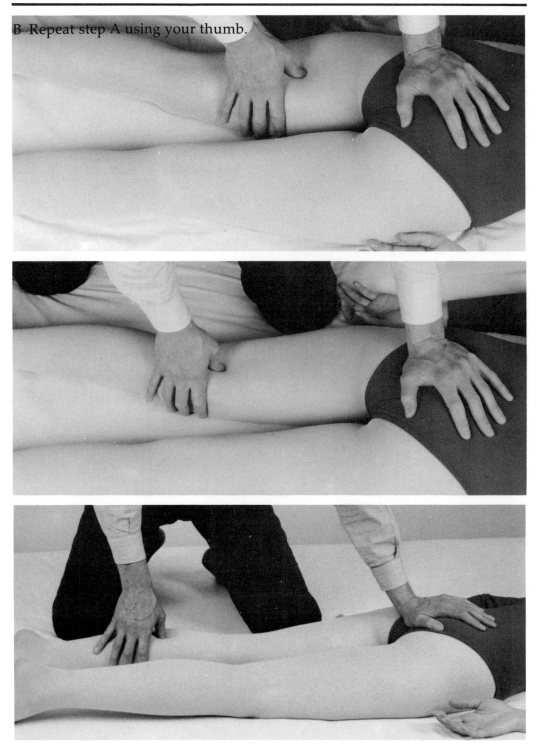

C Repeat step A.

If you feel uncentered when working on the calf, move the support hand down to the area right above the knee.

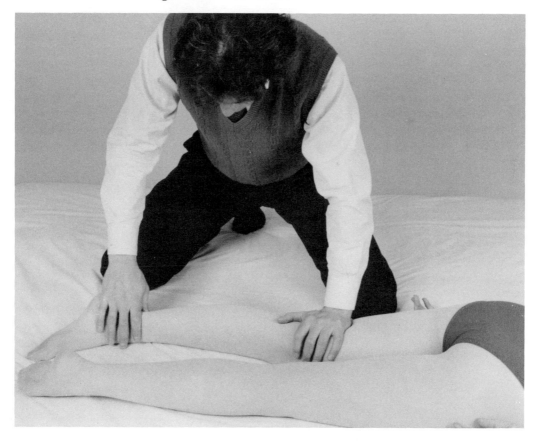

3 Lift the foot so that the leg bends at the knee.

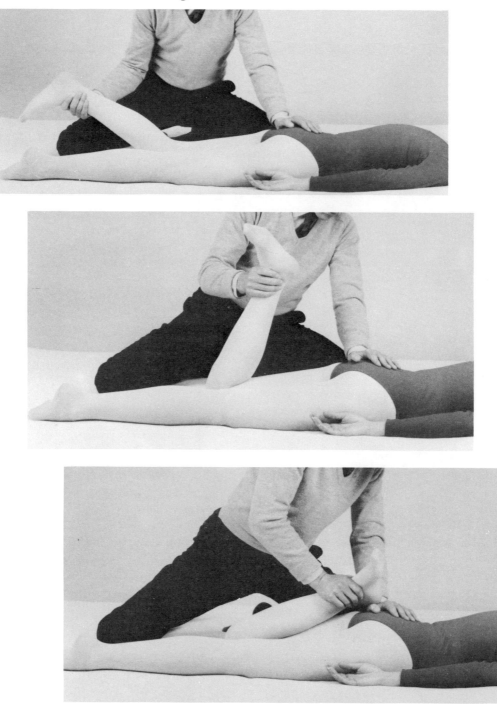

Gently move the foot towards the buttock, being conscious of the leg's stretching capacity. Gently drop the foot back to the floor.

4 Sitting in seiza, lift and rest the foot in your lap.

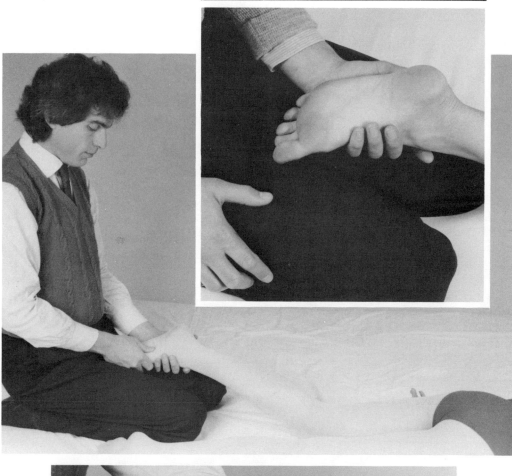

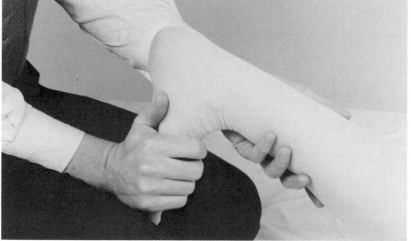

A Stretch the foot to extend the Achilles tendon.

B Roll the knuckles over the entire bottom of the foot.

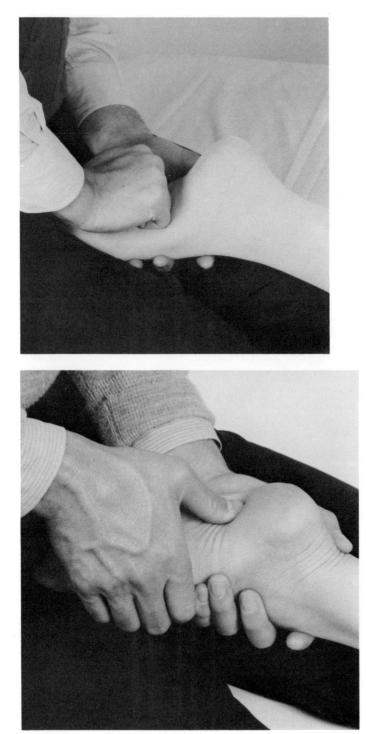

C Give thumb pressure in a line from the heel to each toe.

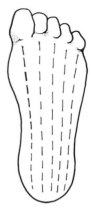

D Stimulate the point in the center of the foot by sinking in, holding, then vibrating slightly. This is Kidney #1, *Yu Sen, "Gushing Spring"* and is useful for reviving a person who blacks out or is knocked unconscious.

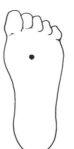

Kidney #1, Yu Sen

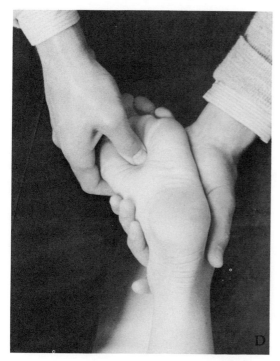

E Squeeze around the base of the small toe. Rotate the toe, then gently pull it outwards. You may hear a cracking sound which means that built-up energy has been released. Repeat on each toe.

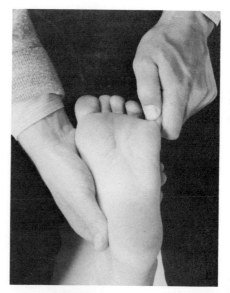

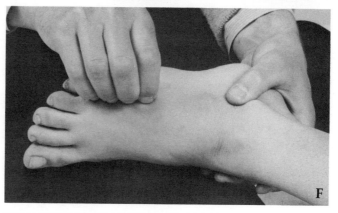

F Using your fingers, squeeze in between the metatarsal bones on the top of the foot.

5 Bend the legs, bringing the feet towards the buttocks. Check and see which foot goes closer to the buttocks.

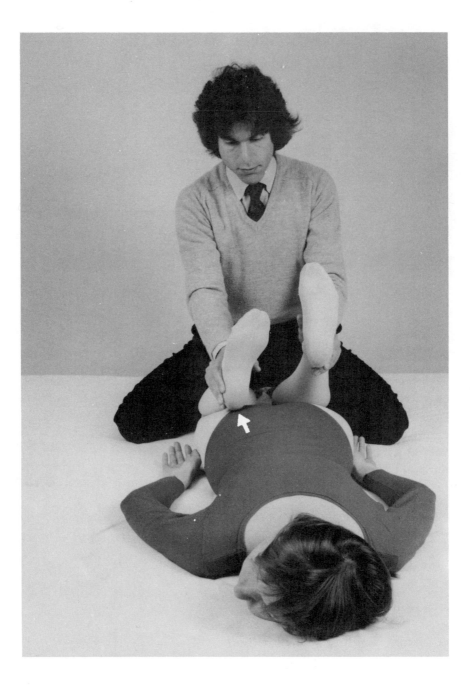

A Cross this foot under the other foot.

B With the legs still crossed, bend them towards the buttocks. Hold for several seconds until you feel the receiver's back and thigh muscles relax slightly into the position. Gently release.

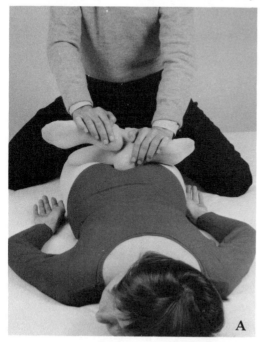

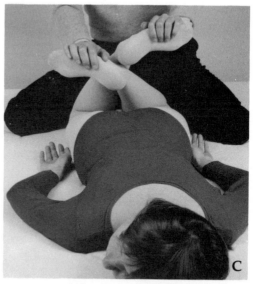

C Reverse the crossed legs.

D Bend the legs towards the buttocks once again; hold; release.

E Uncross the legs and bend them again towards the buttocks, as in Step 5. You will probably notice that the bending capacity of the legs has become more equal. This means that the pelvis has now become more balanced.

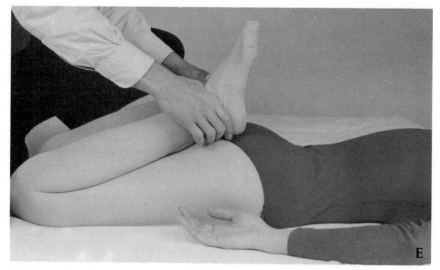

6 Place the other foot on your lap and follow Step 4.

7 Stand on both of the receiver's feet.

    A Give alternating pressure, stepping up and down the feet; avoid stepping directly on the toes.

    B Hold in one position and shift weight back and forth from left to right several times: repeat in various areas of the feet.

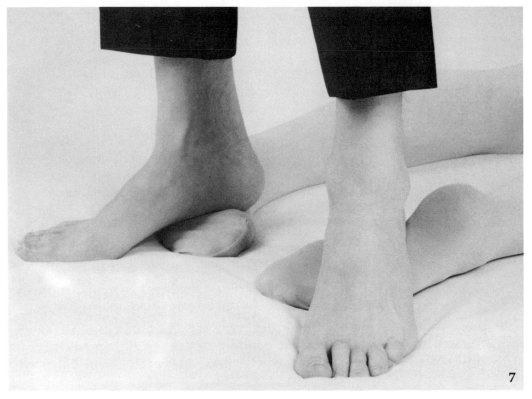

8 Go to the opposite leg; follow Steps 1 and 2.

9 Finish by sitting quietly next to the receiver with your hand placed securely on the small of their back.

Changing Positions

Changing the receiver's position is a very important part of treatment. We should approach this crucial point carefully. The average person exists from day to day in a condition of excess tension. Therefore, even if they have become partially relaxed by the first part of treatment, a call for their own motivated action brings the tight, restrictive condition right back. Watching animals gives us good examples of how to make the change. They stretch slowly, gradually assuming movement as they turn over.

Do not overlook this transition as an effective part of treatment. As with many simple applications like stretching, rocking or gently bouncing the body, we tend to overlook their effectiveness in favor of more complex technique. Carefully guiding the receiver during transition of position maintains continuity and is another way of bringing them to consciously realize that they have 'let go.' When assisting the receiver, encourage them to begin slow movement on the outbreath and physically guide the change with your hands, arms, and body. Turn the receiver over so that they are lying on their back.

Arms and Hands

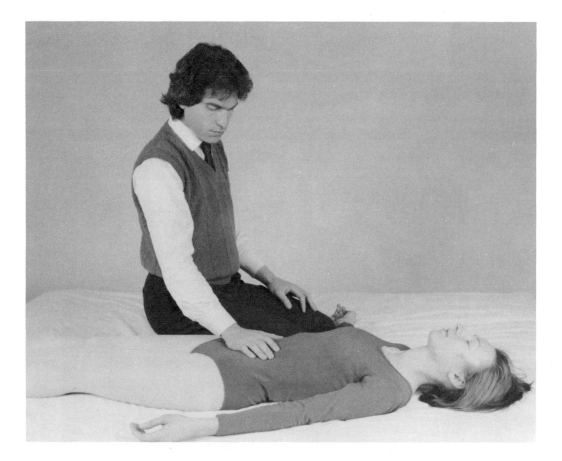

1 Begin by placing your palms on the receiver's shoulders. Bring your weight forward and give pressure.

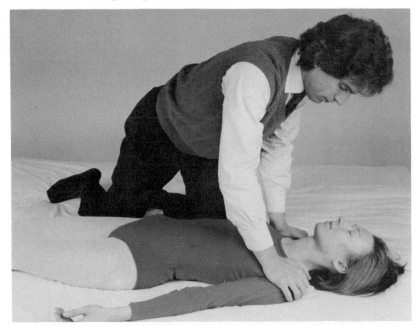

2 Hold one palm on the shoulder and with the other hand give a squeezing, kneading, rolling motion, as in Legs and Feet, Step 1.

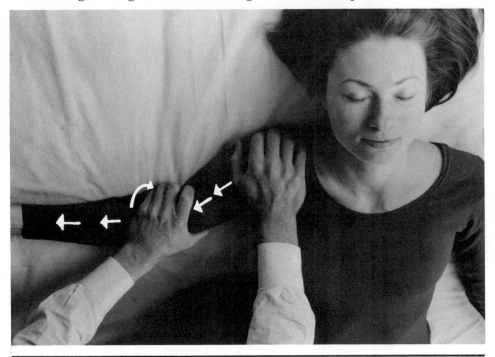

3 Continue to hold a support hand over the shoulder. Give holding pressure with the palm of your other hand down the inside of the arm. Remember to be aware of the sensation under both hands at the same time.

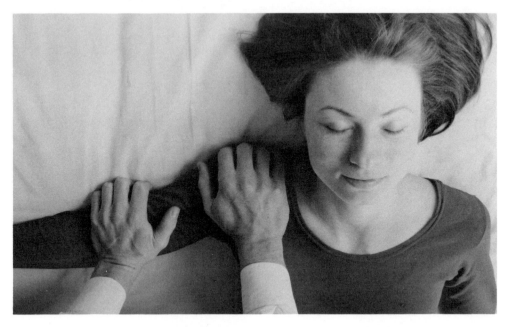

A Thumb down the center of the arm.

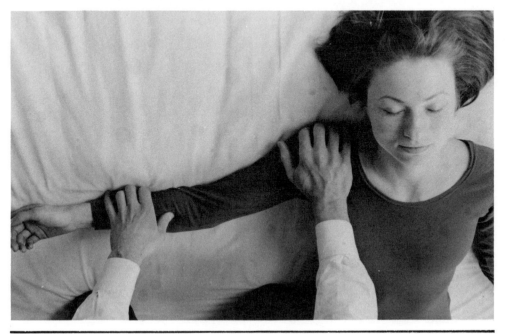

B Palm down the arm again.

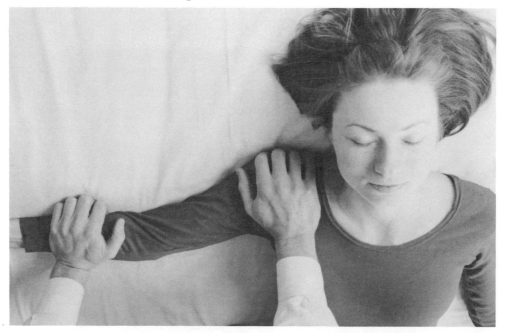

4 Gently stretch the wrist to its maximum. Do this in each direction. The wrist and all other joints can be major places where energy stagnates. Hold these stretches and allow energy to begin moving through to the hands.

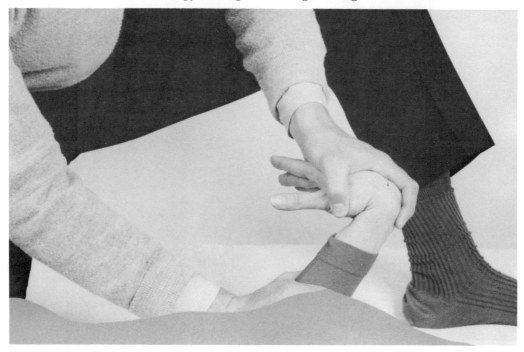

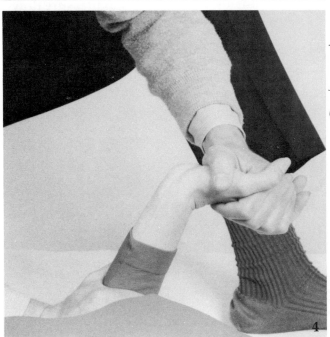

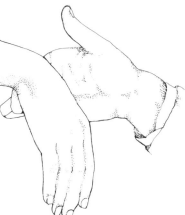

The palm faces down. The underside of the wrist rests on the index finger of each hand. The thumbs roll over the bones on the upper side of the wrist.

5 Quickly flick the wrist back and forth. You may hear a cracking sound which shows calcification and crystallizing of stagnated energy.

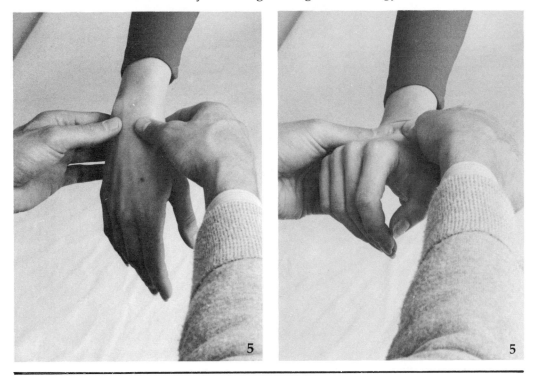

6 Open the receiver's palm with your pinkies, and give thumb pressure down the center three times.

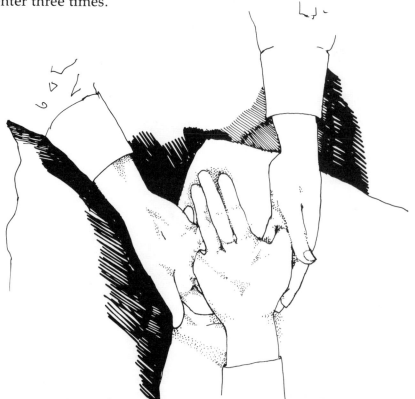

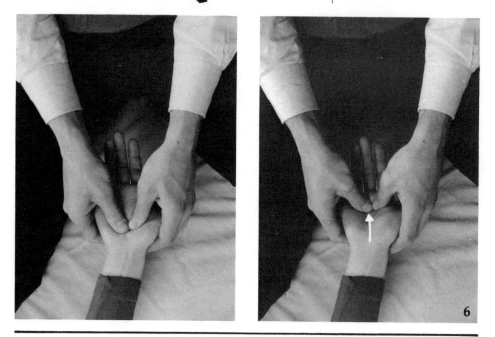

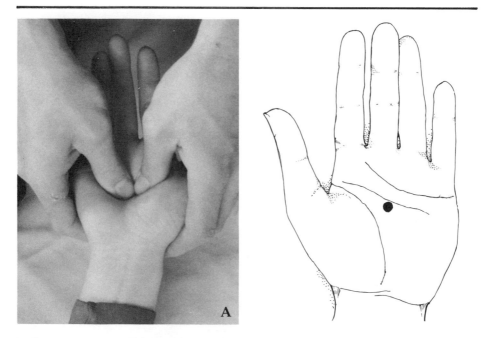

A Give pressure right in the center of the palm. Hold and then vibrate three times. This point is Heart Constrictor #8, *Ro Kyu, "Palace of Anxiety"*.

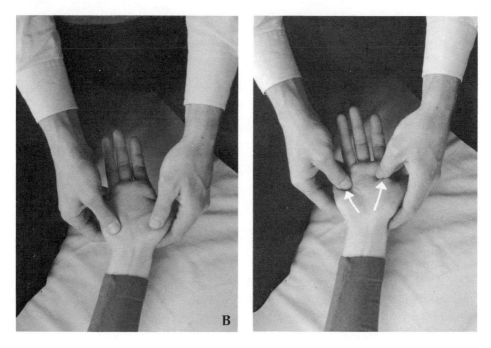

B Give thumb pressure down the outer edges of the palm.

7 Turn the hand over and give thumb pressure at the top of the soft, webbed place between the receiver's index finger and thumb. This point is Large Intestine 24 or *Go Koku, "Meeting of Mountains."*

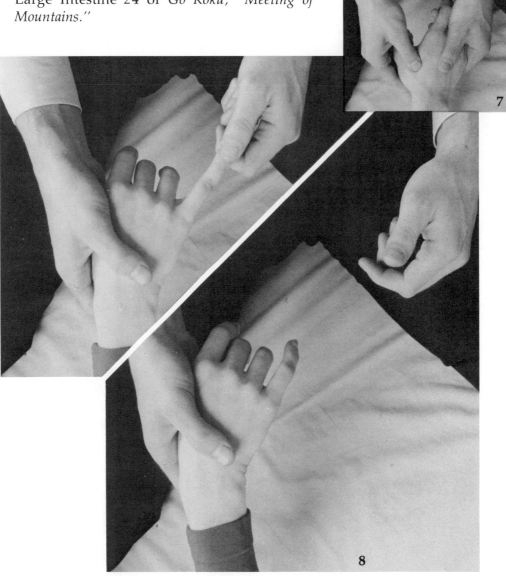

8 Firmly squeeze each flange of the pinky.

  A Rotate the finger and briskly snap it as you let go. This sends a charge into the meridian system which correlates with that finger. (see Diagnosis, page 196).

  B Repeat with each finger.

9 Firmly squeeze the entire hand for several seconds.

10 Move round to the outside of the arm. Hold the support hand at the receiver's wrist. Give palm pressure up the outside of the arm.

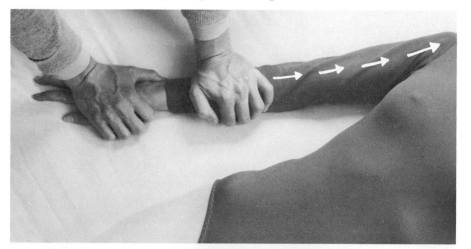

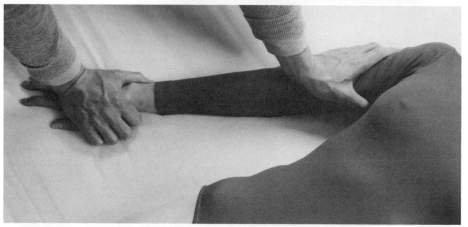

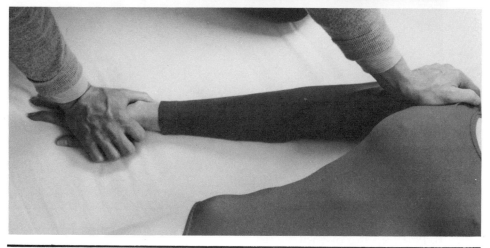

A Thumb up the center of the arm.

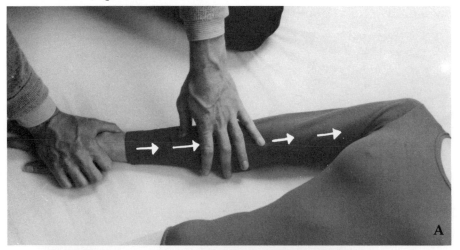

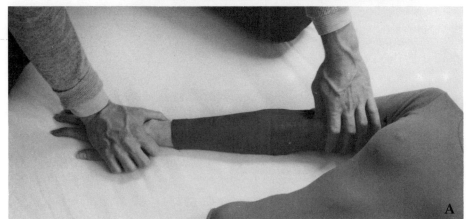

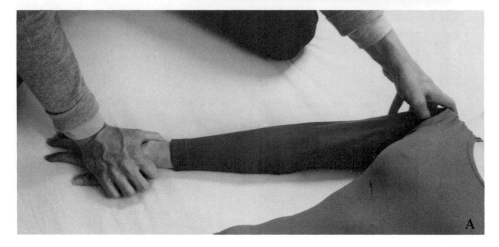

B Palm up the outside again.

11 Holding the receiver's wrist, gently stretch the arm over the head. This is done by rocking back. As you should with all techniques, be aware of how this might feel to the receiver. Experience what they experience during each phase of the treatment. Allow this stretch along the side of the body to open up gradually.

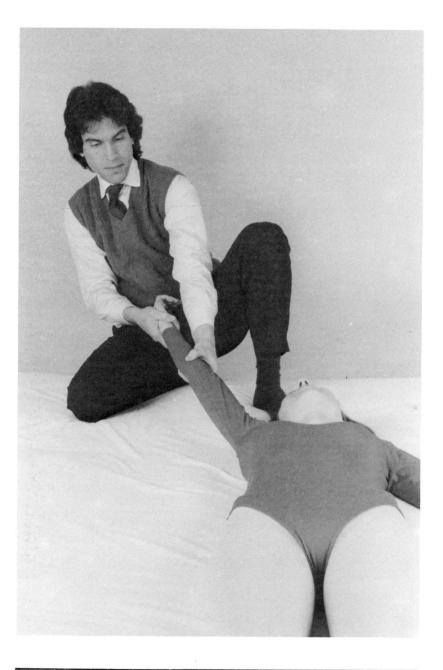

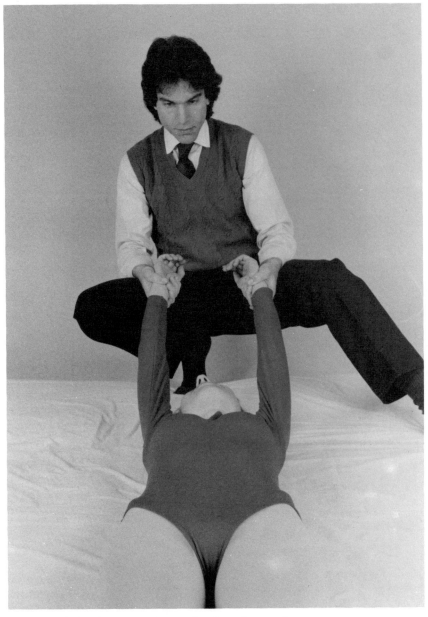

A Stretch both arms above the head together.

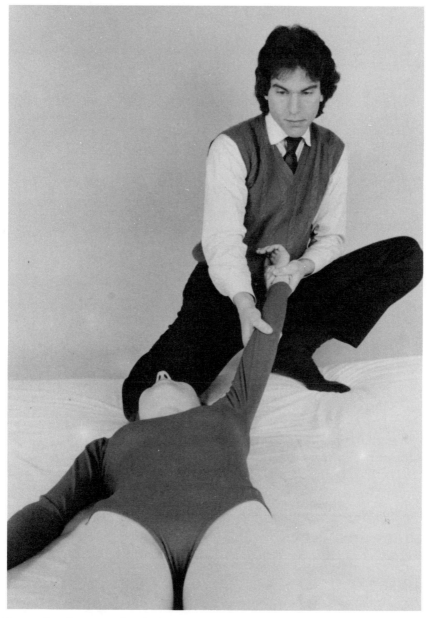

B Drop the first arm back down to the side and then stretch the second arm.

12 Move round to the second arm and repeat Steps 2 — 10.

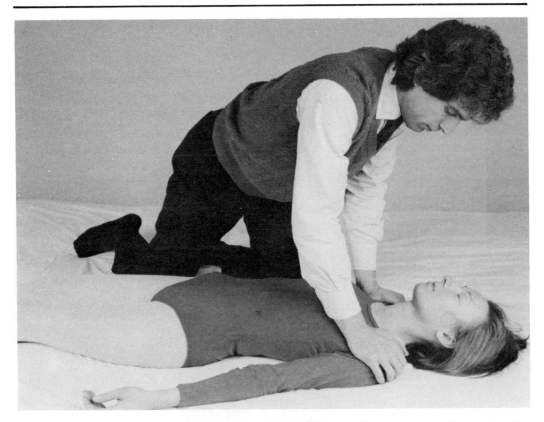

13 Place your palms over the receiver's shoulders and assess any change in the overall feeling, as in Arms and Hands, Step 1.

14 Sit beside the receiver and focus your attention in the hara. Briefly tune into the sensation they are now experiencing in the upper part of the body. You will sense that they are lighter and that energy is now actively traveling throughout the entire area on which you have just worked.

Shoulders and Neck

SHOULDERS

1 Guide the receiver into an upright position, supporting them on the back and neck.

Many people have difficulty sitting this way due to troubles in the intestines and/or reproductive organs. If so, change the angle of their back by propping them up on a pillow. This will allow them to sit with a straight spine. It is very important that the receiver is relaxed and comfortable. If you feel that the receiver is struggling or becoming tense in any position or during treatment in general, modify the position or find some alternative method of supporting them.

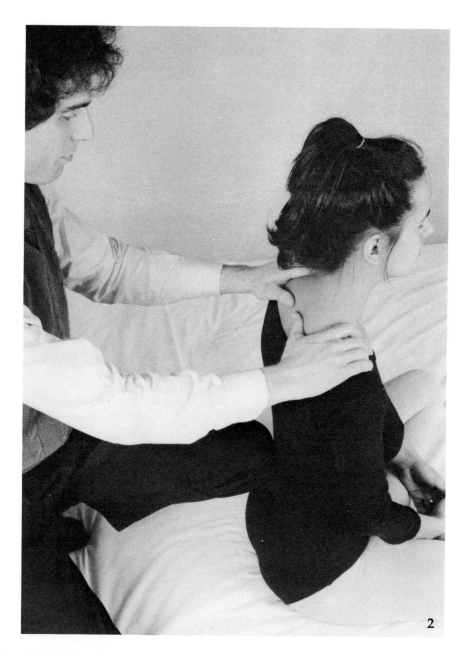

2 Kneeling behind the receiver, hold both hands on their shoulders. Assess the overall condition of energy and muscles.

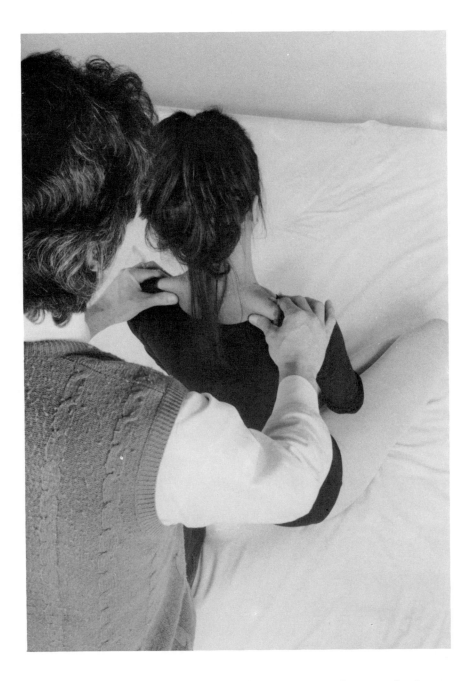

3 Knead both shoulders at the same time by squeezing the muscles between the thumb and fingers. Start out gently and become as vigorous as their capacity will allow. Then alternately knead one shoulder at a time, moving from the base of the neck toward the arms.

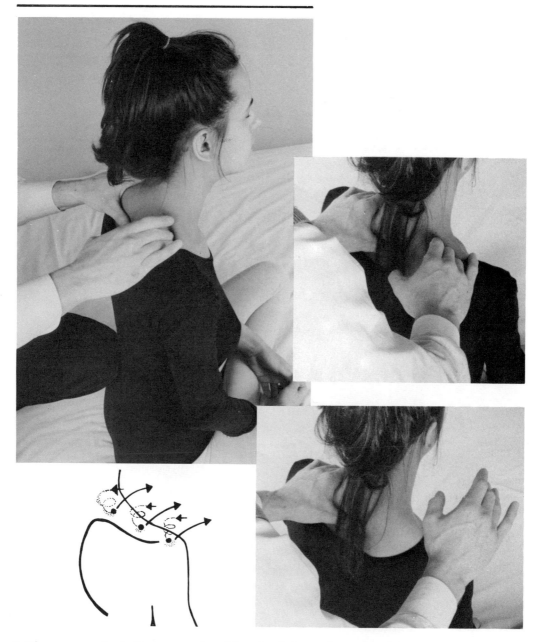

4 If you can feel that one shoulder is tighter than the other, begin the next technique on the looser of the two.

    A Starting at the base of the neck, make a spiralling motion with the fingertips. Start with the least amount of pressure at the surface; gradually go deeper and deeper; then release suddenly. Move to the next point, toward the top of the arm, and repeat.

    B Repeat on the other shoulder.

5 Knead both shoulders again.

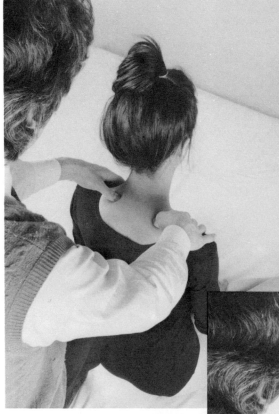

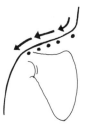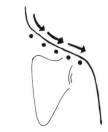

6 Give thumb pressure on the shoulder, holding each point. Start at the base of the neck and move outward; repeat one to three times.

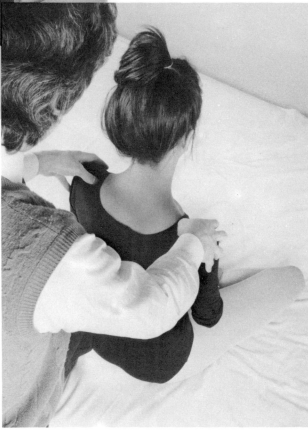

7 Knead both shoulders again.

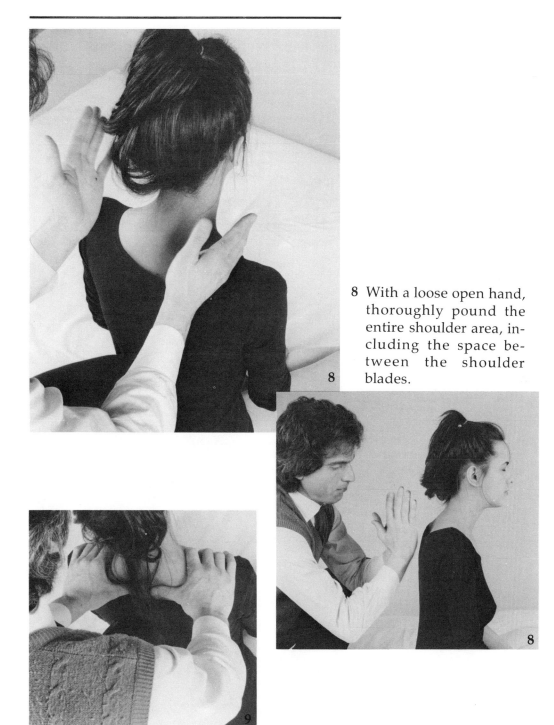

8 With a loose open hand, thoroughly pound the entire shoulder area, including the space between the shoulder blades.

9 Hold your hands gently over the shoulders and assess any changes in their condition.

NECK

1 Support the forehead with one hand and the neck with the other.

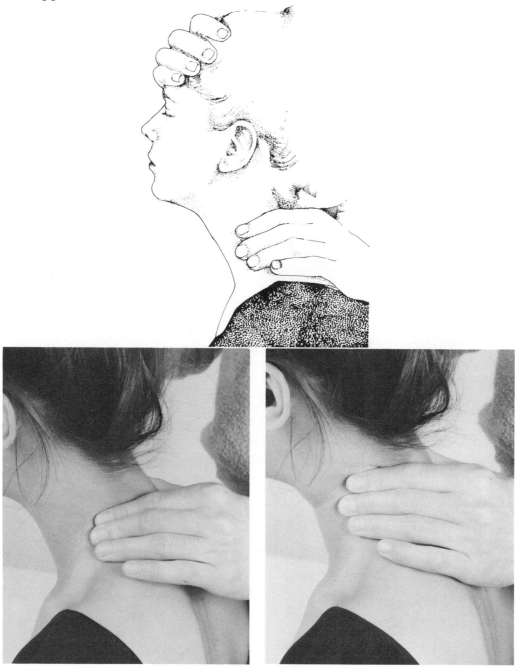

2 Using a squeezing motion *between* the thumb and fingers, firmly knead the sides and back of the neck. Start under the skull and work down towards the shoulders.

3 Roll the fingertips firmly across the muscles on the side of the neck. Again, begin gently and become more vigorous and deep as you gauge the receiver's tolerance. Repeat on the other side.

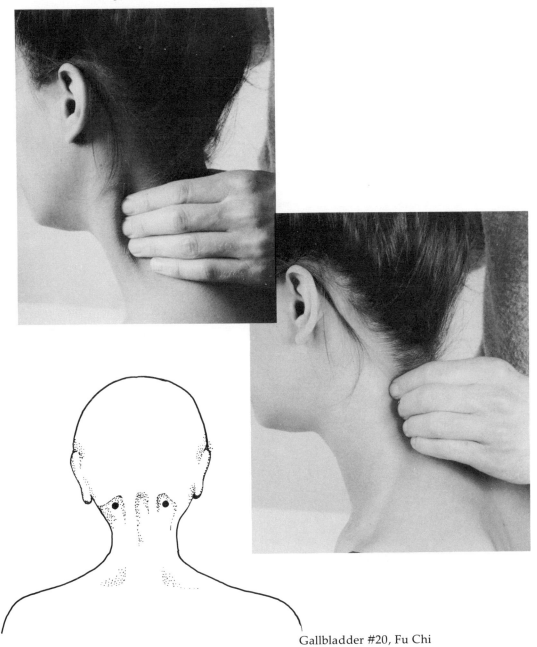

Gallbladder #20, Fu Chi

4 On the side of the head, find the indentation under the occipital ridge of the skull. Place the thumb in the soft spot underneath the bone. This point is Gallbladder #20, *Fu Chi,* "Wind Pond."

A Breathe in together with the receiver as you move the head forward.

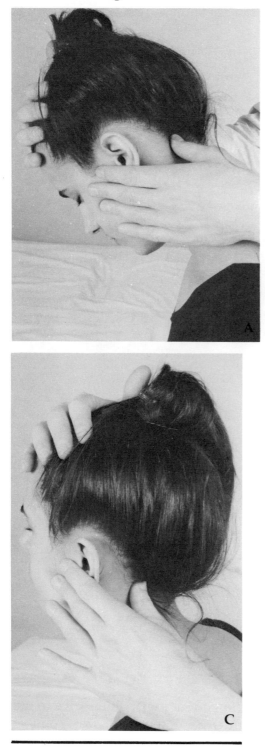

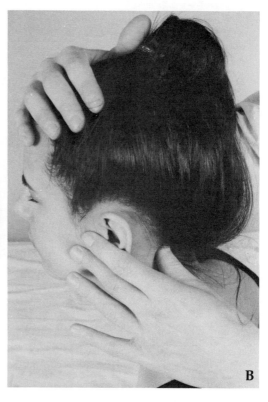

B Breathing out together, guide the head back to the erect position. As you do this, gradually apply firm pressure to the point.
C While holding pressure you can vibrate for added stimulation; repeat one to three times.
D Repeat on the opposite side.

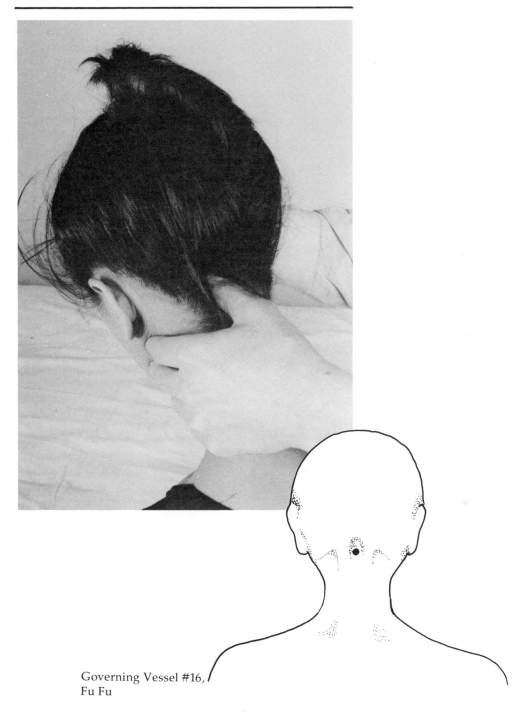

Governing Vessel #16,
Fu Fu

5 Next find the soft spot right in the center between the gallbladder #20 points. This point is Governing Vessel #16, *Fu Fu, "Capital of Wind"*. Place the thumb in this spot. Use the technique described in 4 A-C.

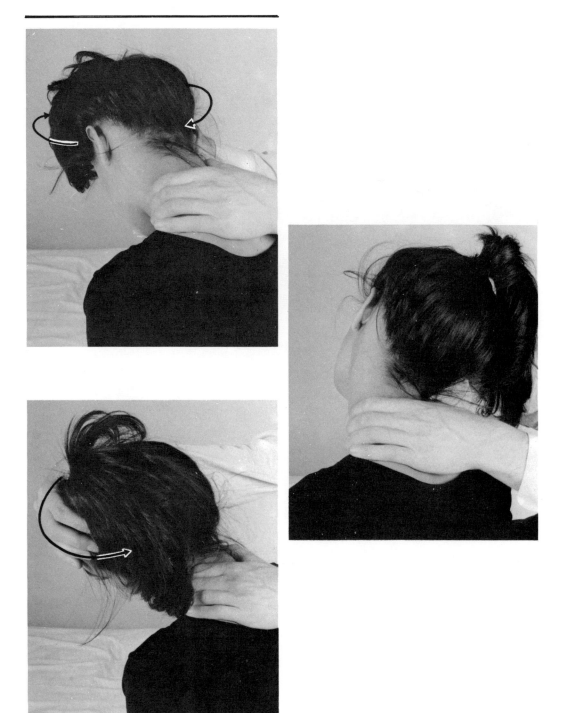

6 Carefully rotate the head through its full range of motion; repeat twice, then rotate again in the opposite direction.

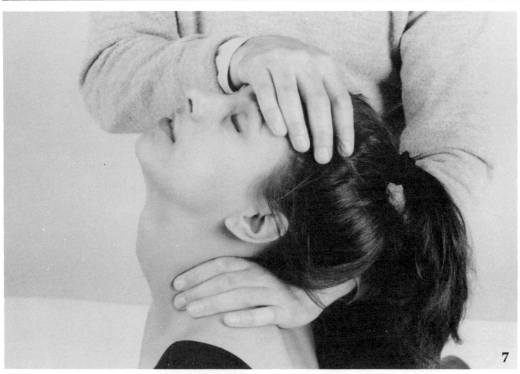

7 Compress the head back and hold.

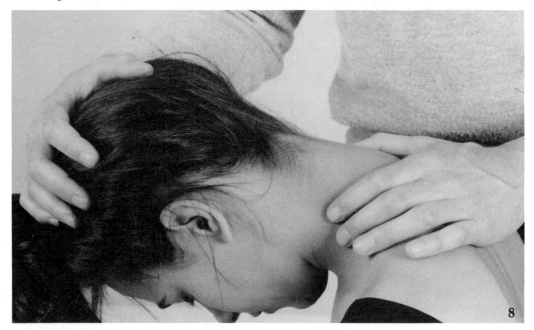

8 Stretch the head forward, opening up the spaces between the vertebrae.

9 Return the head to the erect position.

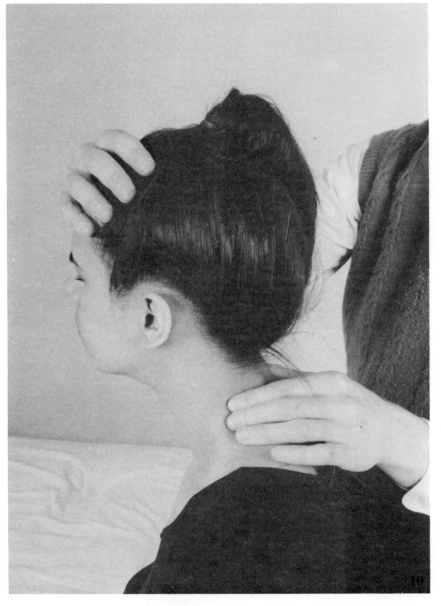

10 Sit quietly supporting the forehead and neck. Hold firmly until you sense a current of energy passing between your hands.

At this point the receiver should feel very light. Slowly remove your hands.

Head and Face

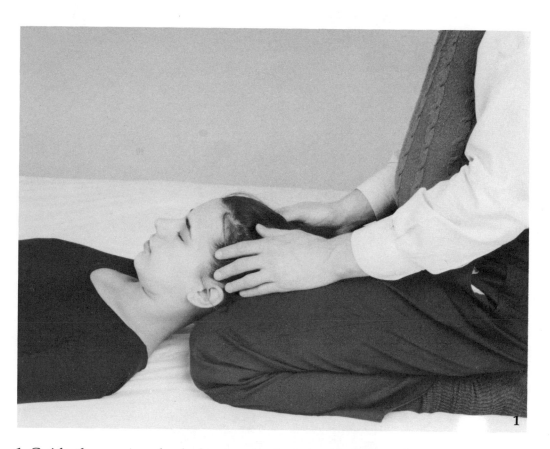

1 Guide the receiver back down onto their back, placing their head on your knees.

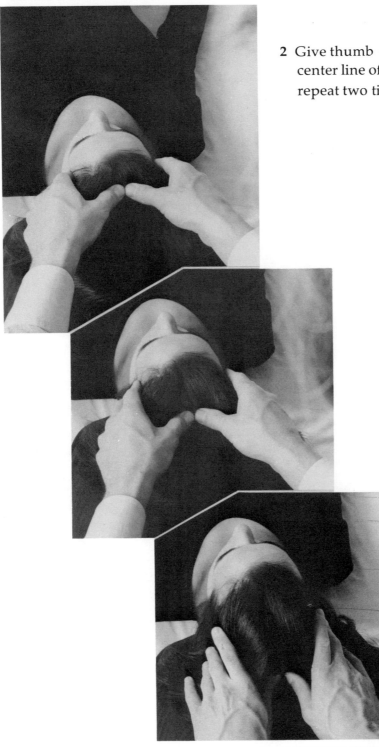

2 Give thumb pressure down the center line of the top of the head; repeat two times.

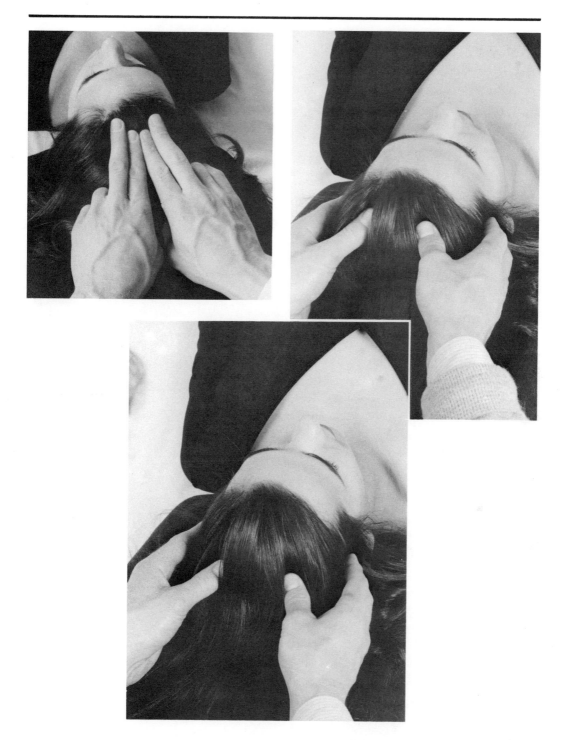

3 Give thumb pressure in a line two fingers' width from the center line; repeat two more times.

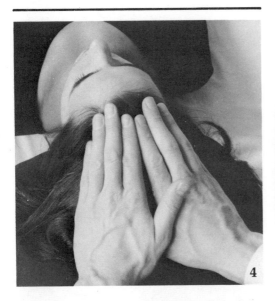

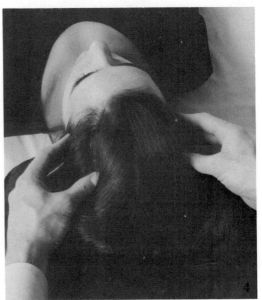

4 Give thumb pressure in a line four fingers' width from the center line; repeat two more times.

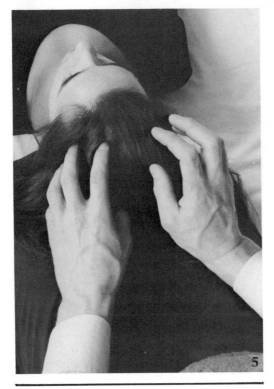

5 Using the fingertips, vigorously tap the entire top of the head.

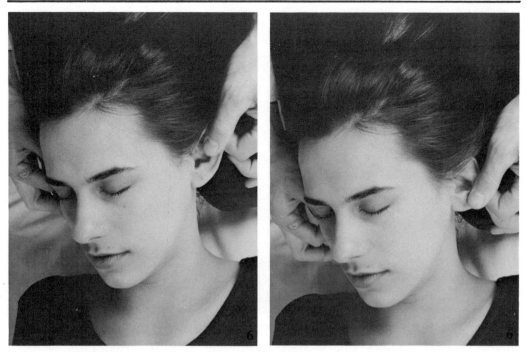

6 Gently pull outwards on the ear lobes. Then repeat around the entire rim of the ears. Do this several times.

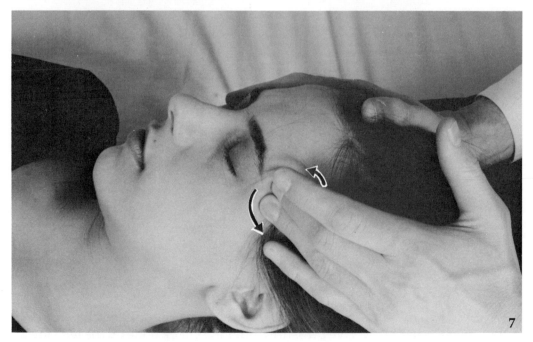

7 Using the middle and ring finger, briskly stimulate the temple area with a rotating movement. Repeat on the opposite side.

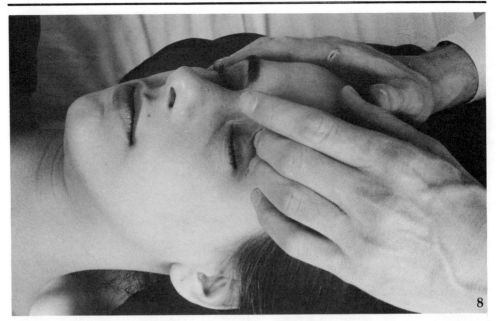

8 Using the middle and ring finger, give pressure along the bony ridge above the eye. Begin at the bridge of the nose and move along towards the outside. Do one side at a time.

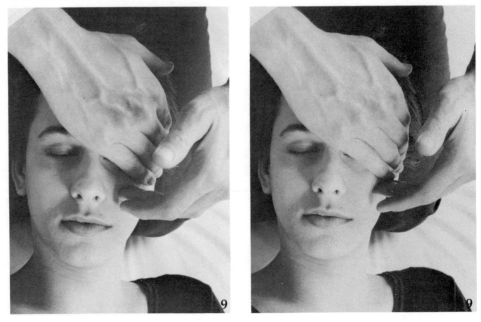

9 Hold your right hand over their left eye. Then, using the middle and ring fingers of the left hand, give pressure under the cheek bone on the left side of the face. Start at the nose and move out towards the ear; repeat one to three times.

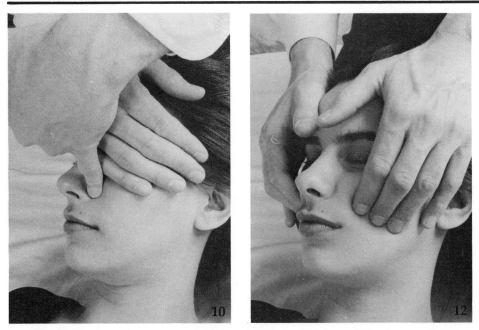

10 Give pressure with the pinky to the indentation at the base of the outside of the nostril.

11 Repeat Steps 9 and 10 on the other side of the face.

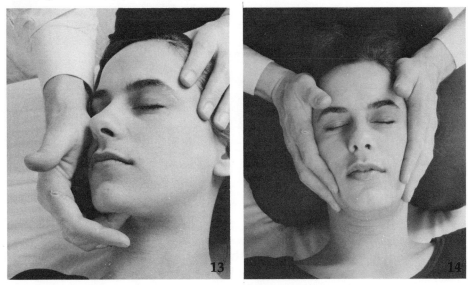

12 Using the fingertips, thoroughly massage the upper and lower gums.

13 Using the middle and ring fingers of both hands, gently give pressure to the soft area under the chin.

14 To complete the shiatsu treatment give pressure with your palms to both sides of the head. Avoid pressure on the ears.

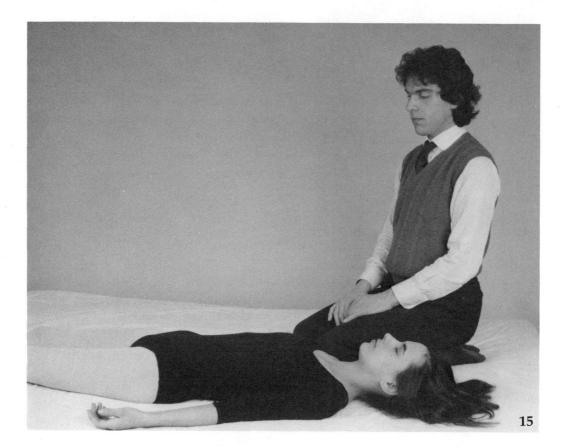

If you gradually and gently release the pressure you will feel a slowly oscillating pulse. If the pulses are uneven, hold patiently. This will then allow them to become more rhythmically even.

15 Quietly suggest to the receiver that they observe how their body now feels from head to toe. Encourage them to release all thoughts and to stay completely relaxed. Move off to the side and sit in seiza. Sense the experience of energy that the receiver is now having.

Rocking Method

The rocking method is used to encourage the receiver to give up conscious control and restriction of their body movement. Rocking relaxes a person due to its relationship to embryonic movement. It recreates a unified and secure feeling that we experienced in the womb and helps to subdue the conditioned ortho resistances developed since birth.

When the receiver is holding and restricting the movement of their body and limbs, their energy is still not moving freely and the deep energy channels are not opened. In this condition it is more difficult for you to help redirect and reorganize their ki flow. When the recipient lets go, opens up and relaxes, many adjustments and changes are possible.

To learn this rocking method first practice it as a treatment itself, systematically moving around the body, rolling and rocking it in different ways, adapting the technique according to the part on which you are working. If you are moving and directing your energy from your hara, this will take no effort at all on your part. If you use muscle strength it will make you tired. As you rock the receiver, you should begin to sense the person's ki moving and rippling in waves throughout their body. This is a very gentle yet powerful technique and encourages the receiver to relax and open up.

When using this method make sure you move each part of the body through its full range of motion. At the same time you should be sensitive to the parameters of each individual's movement so as to allow the person to stay completely relaxed. Most of the time you can create quite a lot of easy flowing motion with very little effort.

If the recipient becomes tense it will defeat the purpose of this method and work against the goal of treatment. Watch the receiver and allow yourself to feel what they are feeling and experience what they are experiencing.

As the body moves in a wave-like motion you may also notice stuck, hard, and resistant areas. This is useful for diagnosing the imbalances of the receiver's energy and influences both the next steps in the treatment and the treatment as a whole. These areas can also show us the organs and meridians involved in the receivers problem. For example:

Indications	*Related Conditions*
stiff thighs	stomach/spleen meridian is blocked or weak.
lack of pelvic mobility.	reproductive difficulty.
stiff heavy shoulders.	lungs are imbalanced.

When using rocking techniques the receiver should gradually allow their body to become limp. If they are still holding, you will feel a resistance to the flow in the movements. If you move the receiver too suddenly or with too much force they will automatically resist. Start with a small amount of motion and gradually work up to maximum movement.

Some of the people we work with are so deeply tense they need to actually learn how to relax their bodies. First try to imply what you want them to do through your intention and the technique itself. If they still resist, guide them verbally and give them some images to follow.

For example:

• Just say   "Please relax", "Let go", "Make yourself limp" or give them the image of making their body limp like a rag doll or a puppet on strings to evoke a sense of looseness.

Feel free to make up anything appropriate in order to achieve this result.

Rocking Technique 1

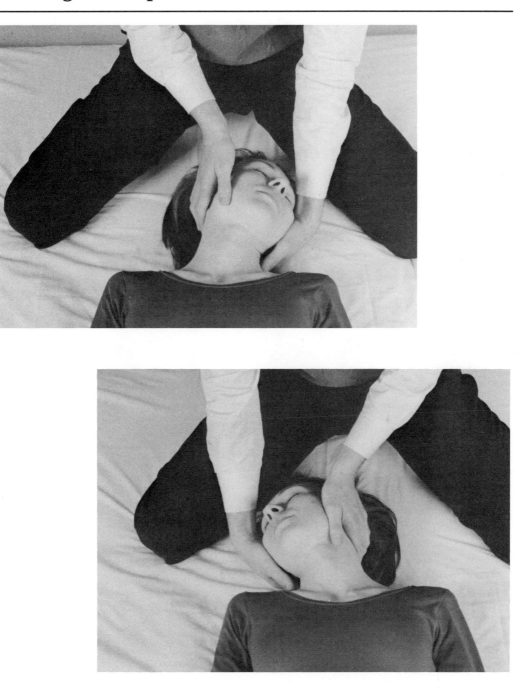

With the person on their back:
A Roll the head between your hands until the head and neck feel loose.

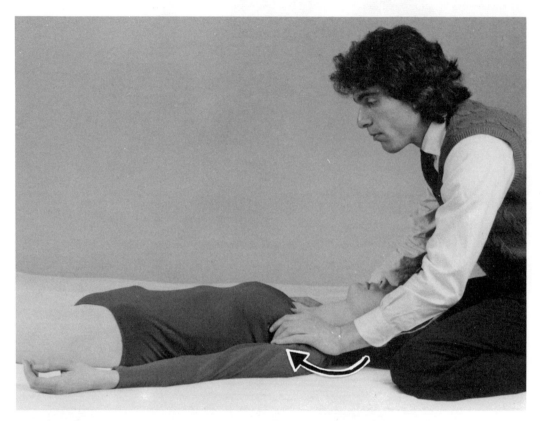

B   Rock the shoulders, directing the ki flow down towards their feet. Move both
    back and forth together, then alternate.

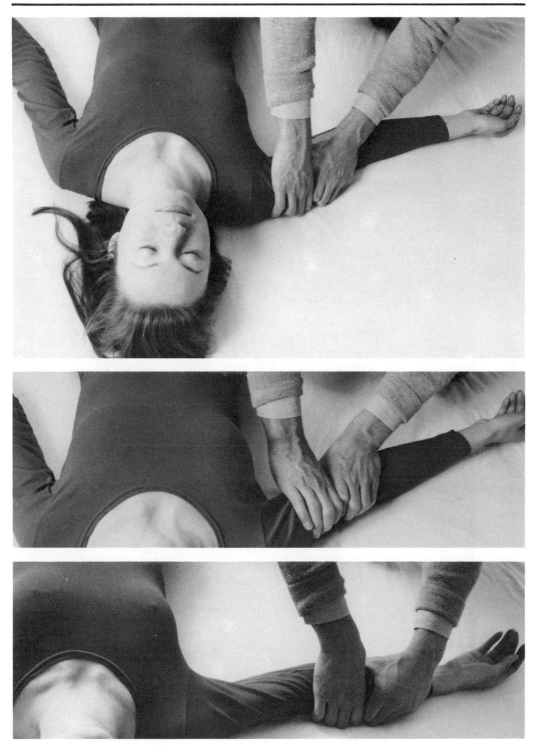

C   Actively roll the arm from the shoulder to the hand.

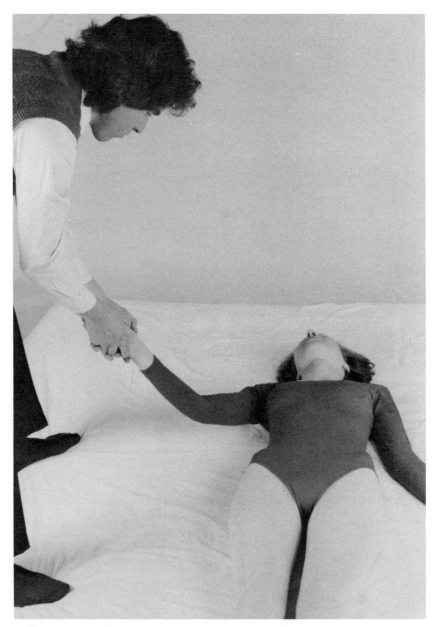

D Hold the hand at the wrist and gently shake the entire arm from the shoulder. Make sure the elbow and wrist are moving and loose. Gently drop the arm.

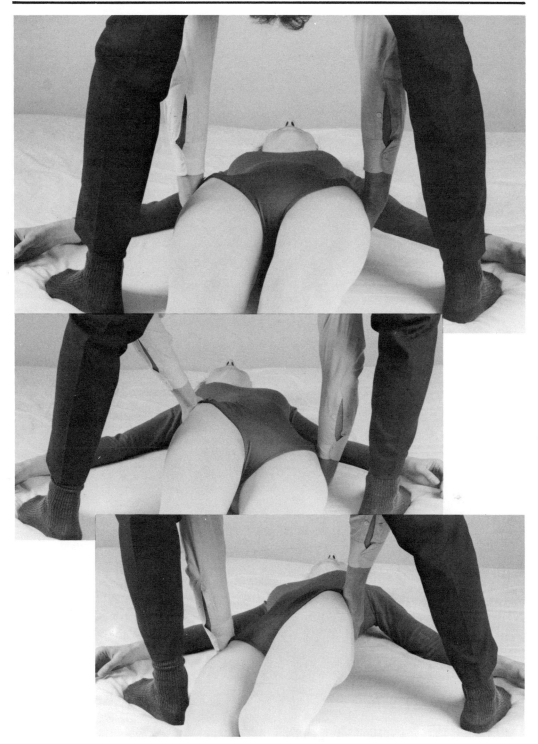

E   Gently pick up the pelvis and roll it from hand to hand.

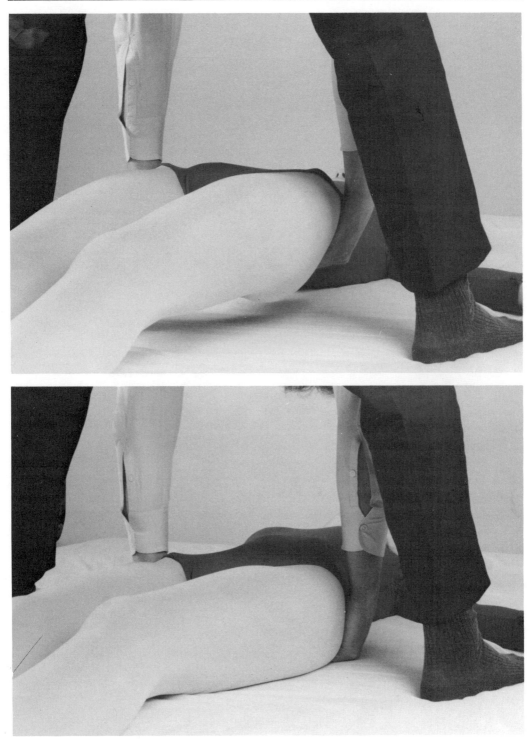

F   Gently bounce the pelvis.

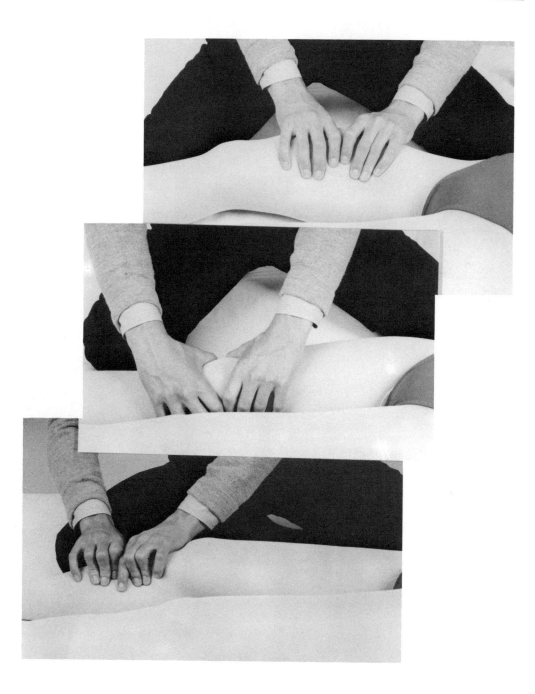

G Roll and knead the leg with both hands, starting at the thigh and moving down to the ankle.

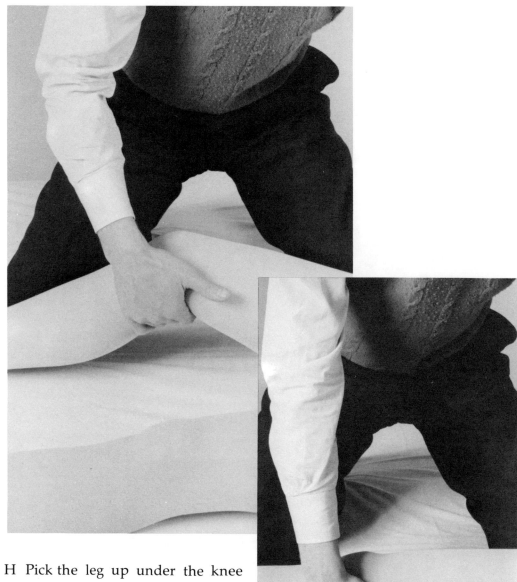

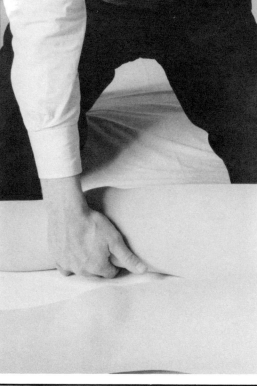

H Pick the leg up under the knee
   and gently bounce up and down.

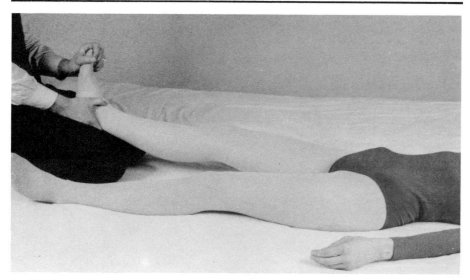

I   Pick up the foot and place it in your lap.

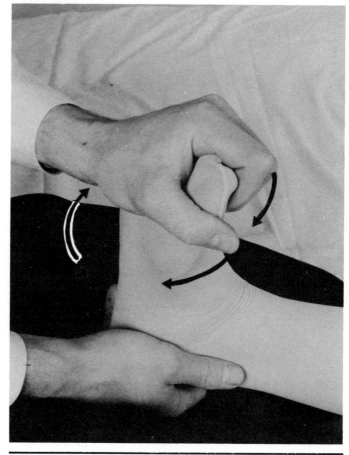

J   Cup the ankle in one hand and, with the other hand, rotate the foot and ankle joint.

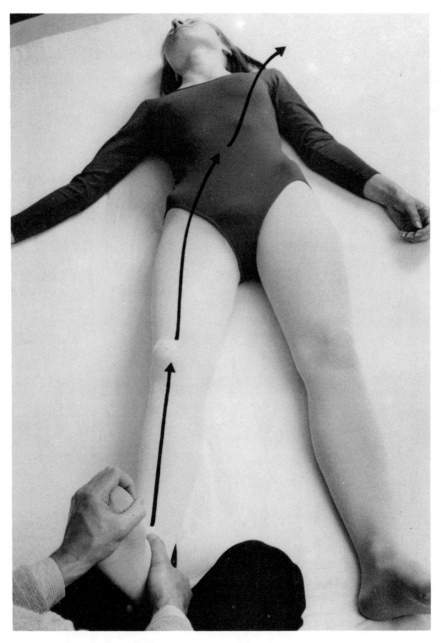

K Notice the line of drive which moves diagonally through the opposite shoulder, including the head.

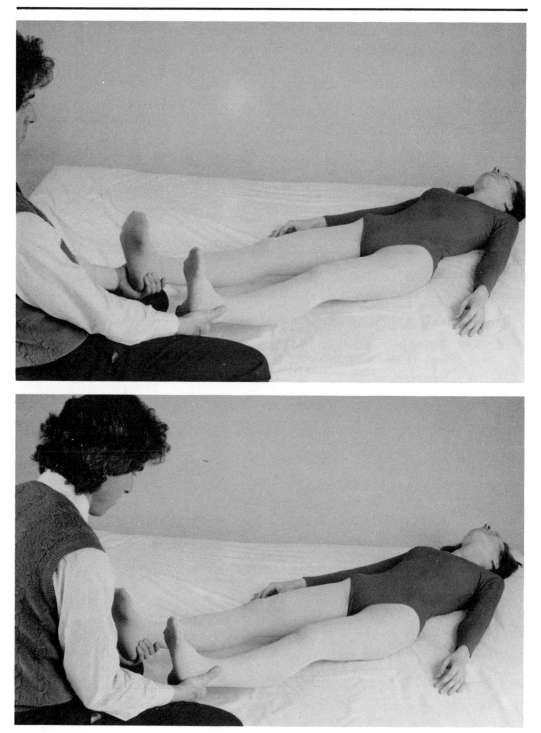

L   Hold both ankles and rock the whole body. Repeat steps A-G on the other side of the body.

Again, start each movement slowly and allow it to build in intensity. Then diminish the intensity, allowing the body to come to rest by itself. Even after the actual motion stops, the receiver will still experience the moving energy as if the body itself were still moving. You should also sense that the receiver is feeling this sensation and you should be able to gauge the activity of their ki flow.

While performing these techniques you should be relaxed and at the same time constantly move from your hara. Always feel as though you are participating in the technique as if you were an extension of the receiver's body. Remember, if you expect their ki to move, yours must also be moving. You are constantly directing and influencing the energy. Be aware at all times of what is happening. Do not let your mind drift to other things. Keep your focus from the hara.

Rocking Technique 2

With the person on their stomach:

A Rock the shoulders together and then with an alternating motion, directing the ki energy down to their feet. Sense the amount of freedom or restriction in the shoulder blades.

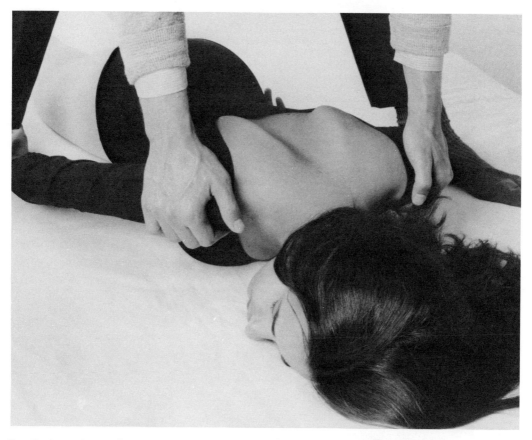

B Pick up both shoulders and gently bounce them. Watch and feel the shoulder blades opening and closing and the movement in the area of the back in between them.

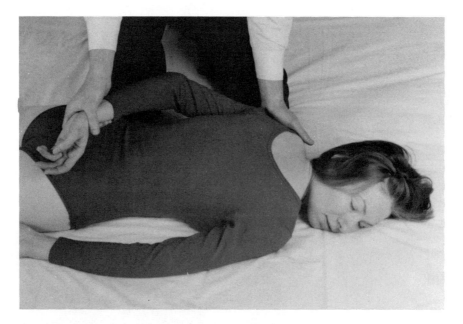

C   Pick up the arm and lay it across the back.

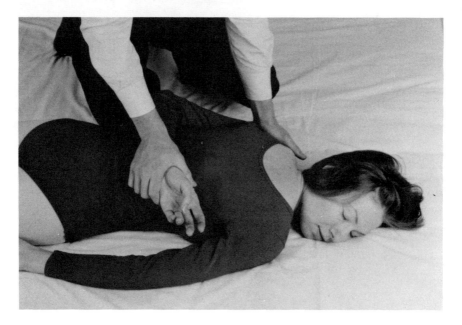

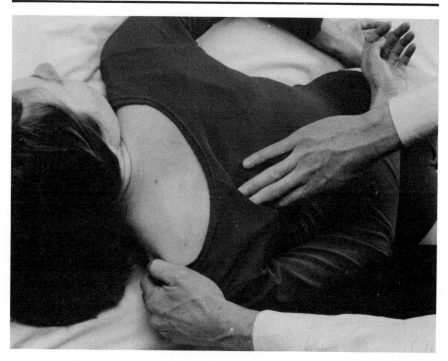

Place one hand under the round of the shoulder and the other with the fingers pointing under the vertebral border of the scapula. Gently bounce the shoulder up and down, moving the fingers under the scapula.

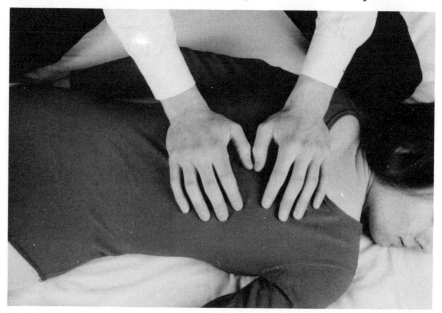

D Roll the back from top to bottom with the hands on one side of the spine and then on the other.

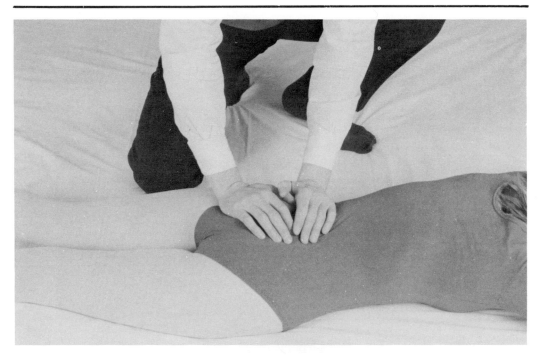

E   Rock the buttocks, gently pushing and rocking. Note that gentle does not mean weak; the movement should be firm.

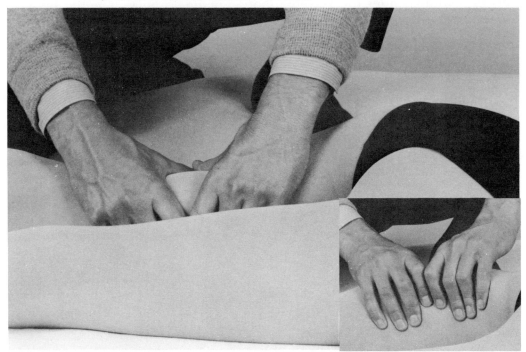

F   Squeeze and knead down the leg while creating a rolling motion.

G Lift and bend the leg at the knee. Bounce the calf, foot and ankle in your hand.

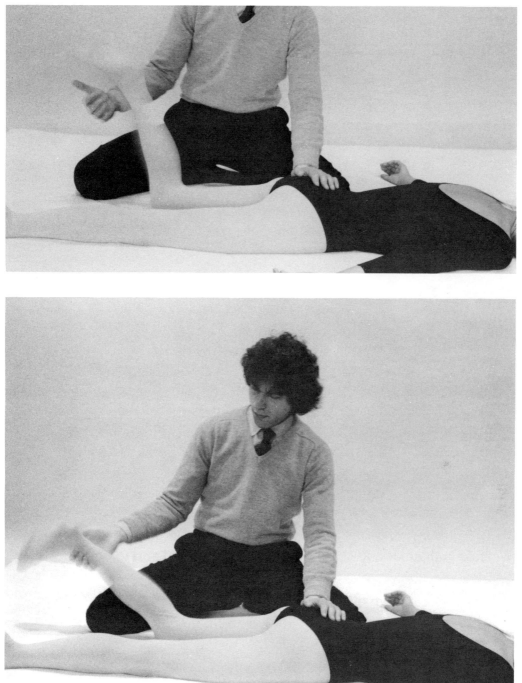

H Hold the ankle in one hand and firmly pump the foot towards the knee. The whole body should move, rocking forward and back.

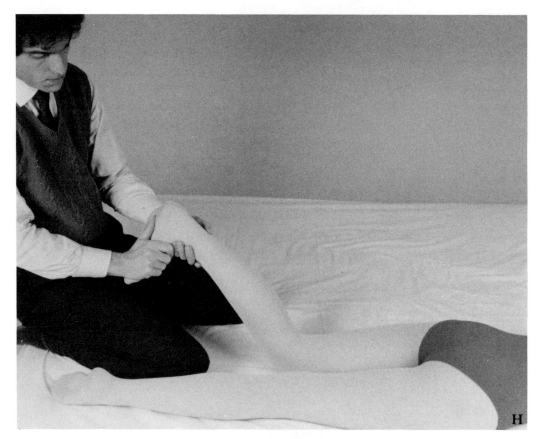

I Hold both ankles. Rock the whole body backward and forward.

Repeat steps working from step G to step A on the other side of the body. Observe and feel the change in the recipient's energy. After practicing for a while you will detect many obvious and subtle changes. For example:

- Distortion in posture from pulling or tightened muscles will even out.
- Misaligned vertebrae will adjust themselves without having any direct force applied to them.
- A tight, spasmed body will loosen and relax.

Once you can perform these routines in a flowing continuous way, the different parts can be incorporated into the Basic Frame treatment. They can be used as a lead-in or transition from one area or technique to the next or when a part of the body seems stuck, jammed and needs encouragement to start ki moving. Rocking can also be used in the complete format presented here and is especially effective when working with someone who cannot relax. Some people are wary of shiatsu, especially if it is their first time having treatment. Being unsure of what it is, they experience an awkward feeling and withhold their trust. Do not hesitate to improvise and adapt your own methods according to what you sense as the receiver's needs. When used as a treatment itself, the rocking method is simple and has a deep and powerful effect on the receiver. It puts them in touch with a state of relaxation and openness that they may not have experienced since being in the womb.

I have had many people laugh and/or cry at the realization that they could open up and let go. So much deep stagnation and holding can be released if we encourage and gently support the person to whom we are giving treatment rather than forcing and causing them pain.

Stretching Techniques

Once you can perform the Basic Frame Outline fluently, please begin to learn and incorporate the following techniques according to their use:

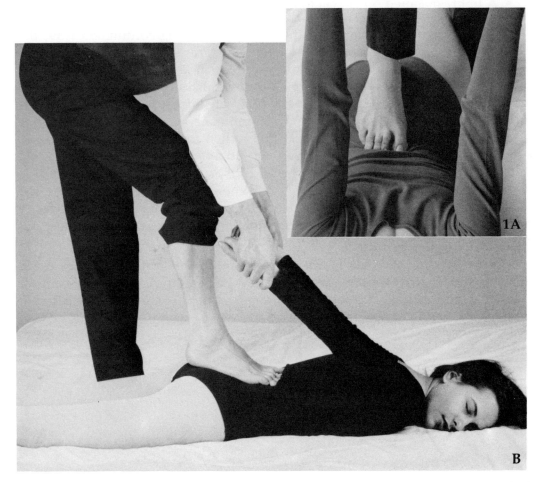

1 A With the receiver lying on their stomach, place your foot in the small of their back with your large toe and index toe straddling the spinal column.

   B Take hold of the wrists.

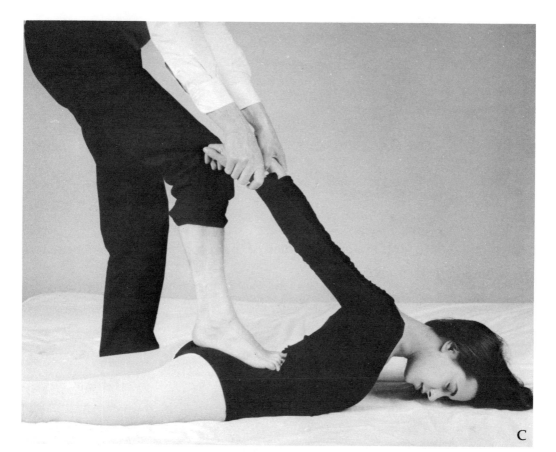

C On the outbreath, arch the back while giving gentle downward pressure with your foot. Make sure the receiver keeps their head and neck limp and hanging forward.

This technique is very good for increasing the flexibility and blood circulation of the spine. It is also beneficial to the intestines as it relieves constipation. Experiment by placing your foot at different places along the spine in order to create a variety of effects.

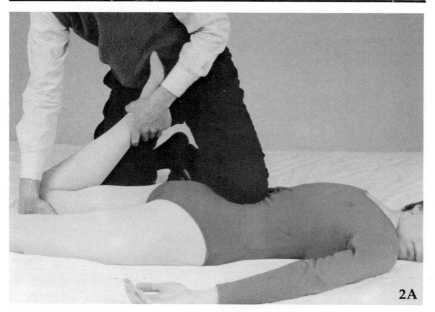

2 A Gently place your knee in the small of the receiver's back, below the last rib.

   B Bend the receiver's knee so that the foot comes towards the buttocks.

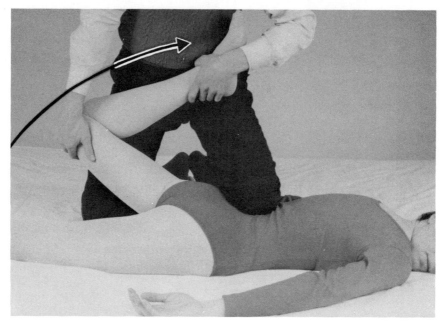

   C Hold the receiver's leg at the knee. On the outbreath lift the leg off the floor.

   D As you lift, gently give downward pressure with your knee. Do three times; repeat on the other leg.

This technique is very good for tonifying and releasing stagnated blood from the kidneys, which are connected to vitality and sexual strength. It also helps to balance the lumbar vertebrae.

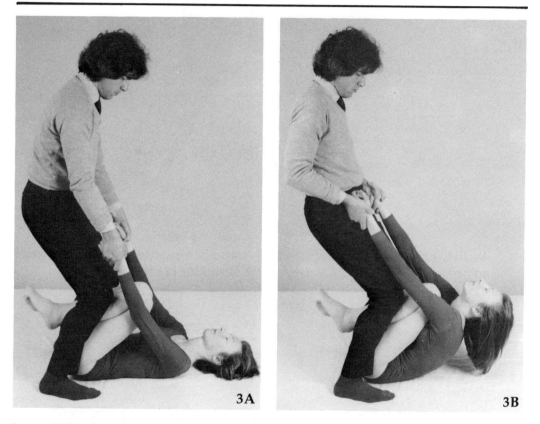

3 A With the receiver lying on their back, bring their knees up as close to the chest as possible. Clasp the arms at the wrist and stabilize their knees by placing your knees up against theirs.

  B On the outbreath, gently bring their chest off the ground. At the same time use your knees to push their knees to their chest.

This technique helps to balance the pelvic bone and releases tension in the groin and middle back.

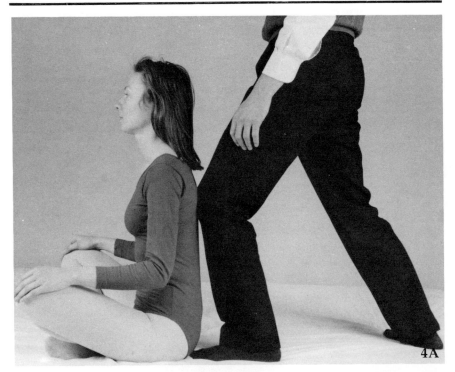

4   A With the receiver in sitting position, stand behind them. Place your knee to one side of the spine, between the shoulder blades.

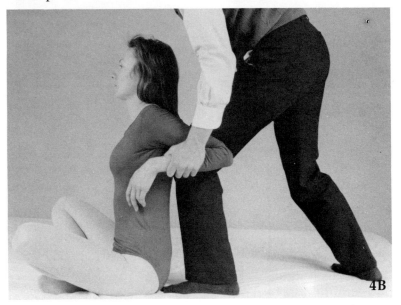

B Holding their arms at the wrist, bend at the elbows; lift the arms and gently pull them backward. At the same time push forward with your knee so that their chest extends out. Do this as the receiver breathes in.

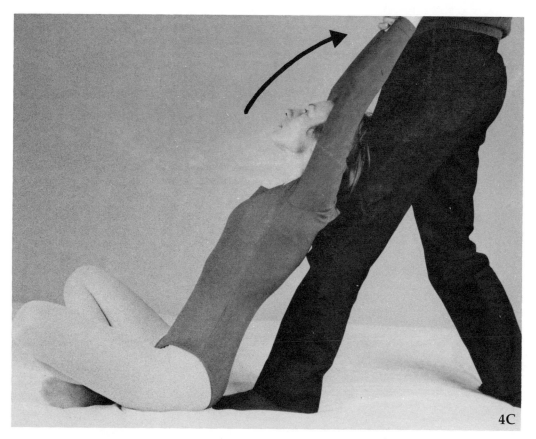

4C

C On the outbreath stretch the arms over the head, both receiver and giver leaning back. Repeat three to ten times total.

This technique increases lung capacity and releases tightness of the neck, shoulders, and chest.

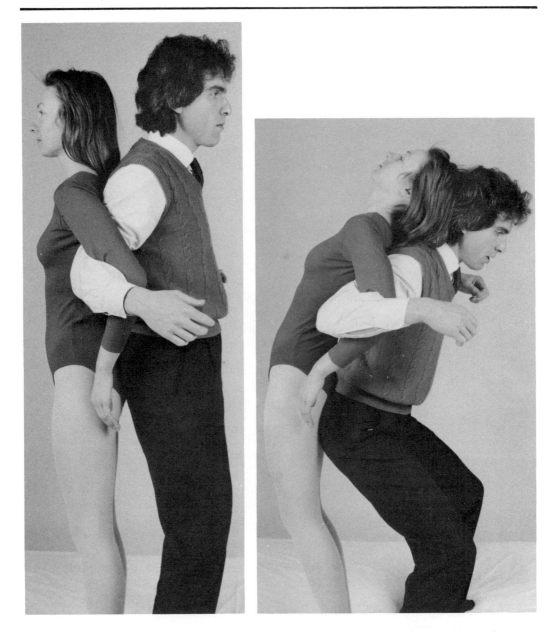

5. A Stand back to back with the receiver and interlock arms. Bend your knees slightly so that your buttocks go beneath theirs.

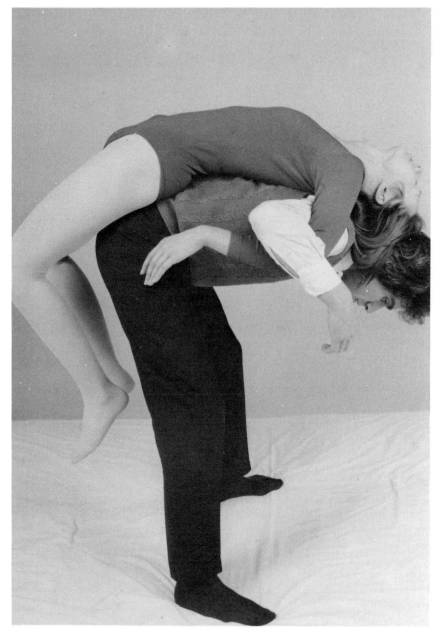

B Bring the receiver up over your back and gently rock them in different directions.

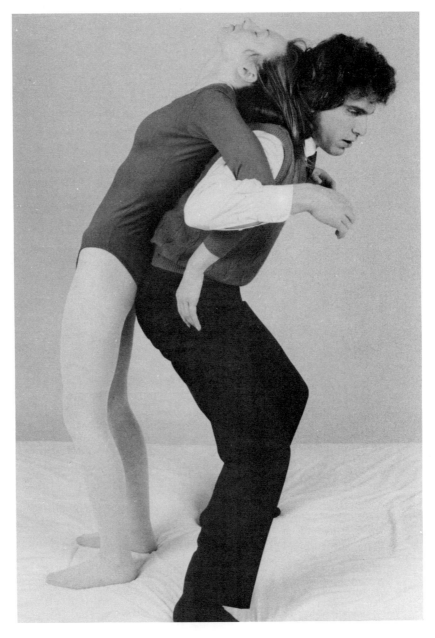

C Gently and slowly, giving careful support, bring the receiver back to the ground.

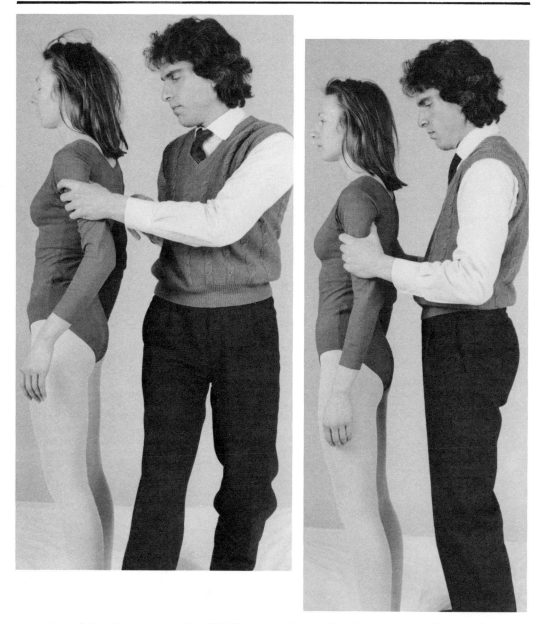

Stand holding them for 15-20 seconds while they regain their balance.

This technique helps the receiver to let go of fear and develop trust. It strengthens and opens the lungs, increases the blood circulation, and gives the receiver a feeling of lightness and peace.

Diagnosis

Many times when people first hear that we are using visual or touch diagnosis to determine a person's health they discount the idea as being nonscientific, fortune-telling, or psychic. They do not realize that they are using diagnosis themselves all the time as a significant part of how they communicate and interrelate with others. We are always consciously or subconsciously making evaluations about the health, character, attitudes, and backgrounds of those around us based solely on what we see and sense as 'gut feelings' or intuition. Often we matter-of-factly express some of these evaluations by saying things like: "Aren't you feeling well?" or "You look tired." We may inquire about someone's health with comments like, "You look a little peaked," or "You look green around the gills." We might judge someone's emotional condition by commenting, "You seem happy," "You look depressed," or "Are you angry?". We may judge someone's thoughts by their expression when we say things like "Don't you believe me?" or "What's on your mind?" When we see people that we do not know we often calculate their ethnic background, religion, socio-economic status or generally the type of person that they are. Simply becoming aware of, identifying, and assessing these impressions are all forms of diagnosis.

Diagnosis, in its true dimensions, extends out to assessing the total experience of a person's life and makes apparent the influence of their ancestors, parents, teachers, and relationships. Diagnosis also considers the movement and effect of the natural and social environment. This enables us to understand how our surroundings influence our past and present condition as well as helps us make decisions and judgements in our daily lives.

The ancient Chinese organized these evaluations and developed a highly refined system of character and health diagnosis based on seeing, smelling, hearing, and touching. Most of the time this diagnosis is more accurate than current systems which deal mostly with symptoms and conditions. It seeks out and exposes the causal factors which are a collation of the person's total past involvements on all levels of their life. It makes visible the future direction of their health and the potential for creating happiness. This enables us to see problems and difficulties that are beginning to develop and gives us the opportunity to use preventative measures to redirect their course. Healing methods used during the stage where difficulty is developing are simpler, easier, and more harmonious with the body and life process than those measures necessary once the problem has manifested. Health problems like kidney stones, arteriosclerosis, cancer, senility, schizophrenia, etc., can be seen long before they actually become activated. This gives the patient plenty of time to change those aspects of his or her life that are contributing to the development of the sickness.

Although we may initially study diagnosis to evaluate health conditions and determine the course of our treatment, in the long run we realize that it is an art form and a lifetime study. Diagnosis gives us an insight and an understanding of nature and creates a deeper, more satisfying, and more complete communication between individuals. It also encourages greater harmony and cooperation in our composite form which we perceive as society.

This section presents a starting point and simple guidelines for the study of diagnosis in conjunction with shiatsu.

How Diagnosis Works

There are two main areas of diagnosis: Constitution and Condition.

Constitution

The time we spend in the womb from conception to birth determines our constitutional qualities. These are set structural formations, tendencies, and characteristics created from the original quality of our parents' reproductive cells and the influence of our mother's diet, activities, and thinking during the nine-month gestation period. Our constitution is also the sum total of all the ancestral and environmental backgrounds from which we emerge.

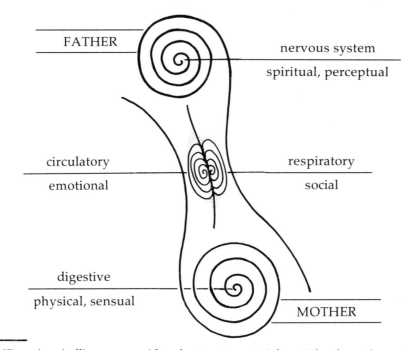

Figure 47 — A spirallic energy gridwork attracts material particles from the mother's blood, creating the basic body functions of the digestive, circulatory, respiratory and nervous systems.

Heaven's and Earth's force coordinate the movement of energy, creating the basic structural alignment of all materialized phenomena. In the initial stage of embryonic development, the energetic spirallic grid-work created by these forces magnetizes material particles from the mother's blood, thus creating our fundamental systems.

The system dealing with our most yang intake and metabolism is the frontal, downward-moving digestive tract, which governs our overall physical and sensual nature. Dealing with the less yang world of liquids and more centrally placed in the body is our circulatory system which is responsible for the nature of our emotions and impulses. Both of these systems and their expressions reflect the influence of our mother's condition and quality. The respiratory system is more central in the body and handles more yin intake. It is responsible for the exchange between oxygen and carbon dioxide and governs our social nature along with territorial instincts and attitudes. The nervous system, which is located towards the back of the body and develops in an upward direction, coordinates the most yin intake and metabolism. This system receives and dispatches the world of vibrations, governing our spiritual perception, images and thought waves. The nervous system and the respiratory system are connected to the quality and condition of our father. (Fig. 47)

mother	*father*
circulatory system	nervous system
emotional	spiritual
digestive	respiratory
physical, sensual	social

The sections of the face which develop concurrently with the body functions reflect the constitutional quality of the primary systems. (Fig. 48)

Equally proportioned sections indicate balance of activity between the systems. If one section appears larger or more defined, it generally tells us that this area of activity and expression is a more dominant trait. Well accentuated and clearly structured sections show inherent strength, while vague, loose or immature qualities imply weakness.

A person's general constitution is either more yang or more yin and is determined by whether Heaven's force or Earth's force is more dominant. Within the make-up of a person's structure, tendency and traits, there is a myriad of qualities, some of which are more yin and some more yang. A person who is structured more compactly and has square features is more yang. Those with elongated, oval features are more yin.

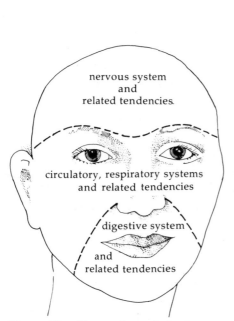

nervous system
and
related tendencies

circulatory, respiratory systems
and related tendencies

digestive system

and
related tendencies

Figure 48 — The sections of the face which develop concurrently with the body functions reflect the constitutional quality of the primary systems. (See page 177)

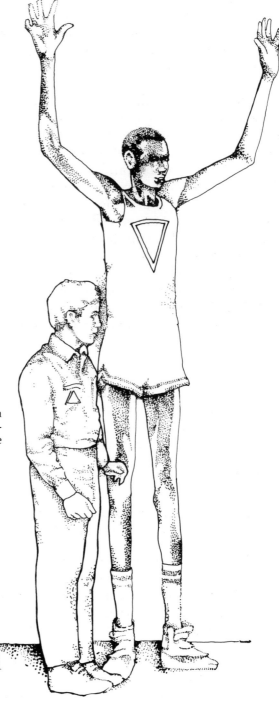

Figure 49 —Yang (left) and Yin (right) constitution.

The following chart gives a general breakdown of yin and yang qualities that are helpful in determining a person's constitution. First use an overall sense to see if it is Heaven's force or Earth's force that dominates. Then compare these secondary traits. Remember that everyone has some of each type of constitutional characteristic that will appear in different areas of their make-up and expression.

Constitutional Qualities

Type	Yang Quality	Yin Quality
movement	active	passive
hair	thick, blond, red	thin, brown, black
eyes	smaller, round, close-set	larger, almond, wide-set
nose	broad, thick	narrow, thin
mouth	small, tight	broad, loose
chin	square	pointed
ears	thick, large	fragile, delicate
shoulders	broad	sloping
bones	heavy	thin
mental/ psychological	practical time oriented structural building monetary	theoretical spatial free form creative imaginative aesthetic
career/life expression	manager builder business politics executive sports	supervisor artist science writer research electronics, computers
environment	spring, summer birth colder climate mountain region	fall, winter birth warmer climate flat lands

Condition

In order to understand diagnosis always keep in mind that the person exists and functions as a whole. The parts reflect the whole, and the whole reflects the sum total of the parts. Our condition, unlike our constitution, which is generally set at birth, is constantly changing under the influence of our eating, thinking, activity, and environment. It shows us the result of our daily lifestyle.

During embryonic development, Heaven's force, moving downward, inwards, and towards the center, has a more dominant influence on the development of the body and the internal organs. Simultaneously Earth's force, which is moving upwards, outwards and towards the periphery, directs the formation of the head and face.

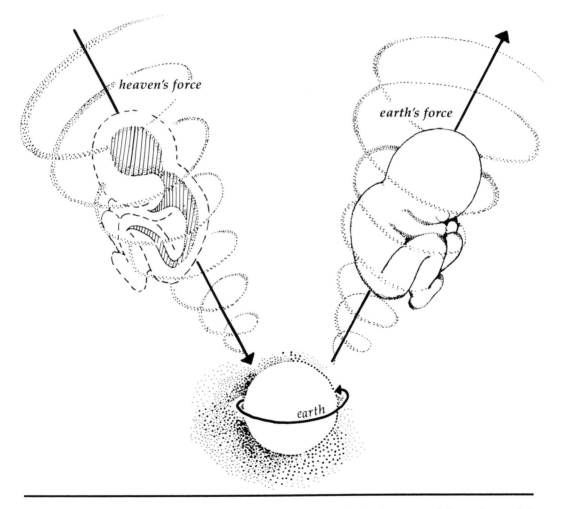

Figure 51 — Heaven's force generates downward and inward development of the embryo while Earth's force generates upward and outward development.

Therefore whatever appears on the inside of the body is reflected in the face; external reflects internal.

If body organs become swollen, hardened, tight, or loose or the body systems become clogged due to unbalanced, excessive dietary intake and lifestyle, the result of this is reflected in the outward appearance of face, posture, and expression. A healthy condition is represented by a bright appearance with resilient, flexible features. Unbalanced conditions that lead to sickness will appear in accentuated skin colors, rough textures or tightness or looseness in the various facial areas. Moles, warts, cyst-like bumps and beauty marks show past sickness and discharge from the organs correlated with the areas of the face in which they appear. They can also show accumulation of proteins, calcifications or the formation of tumors, cysts, and stones.

If we take too much liquid today and develop diarrhea, the lower lip, which corresponds to the intestines, will swell. If we reduce liquids and eat more dry foods, the following day the lip contracts. Too much salt constricts the kidneys, causing a dark hue around the face, tightness under the eyes, and contraction of the lower back. Reducing both salt and drying factors in the diet allows the kidneys to relax and the outward appearances to normalize. Long-term imbalanced intake and habits that chronically overtax the body and systems will begin to distort our features, posture, general expression and appearance. Still, with care and proper diet, these conditions and correlated appearances will normalize. These are just a few examples of the many types of changes that go on from day to day, week to week, and year to year. By monitoring outward appearances and identifying them with what they are related to internally, we can begin to understand and participate in the creation of our health and well-being.

The Facial Map

As you practice studying faces you will begin to recognize the strengths and weaknesses that manifest in a person's changing condition. Use this to confirm what you discover while working through the body giving shiatsu. With experience you will begin to see the foods, habits and environmental factors to which the various conditions relate. (See Fig. 52 Page 188)

Organ	Facial Appearance	Related Conditions
LUNGS & BRONCHI	Sunken cheeks and grayish color.	Poor oxygenation/ lack of facial expression.
	Red swollen cheeks, hardness of texture.	Mucus and fluid deposits, halitosis.
	Broken capillaries in cheeks and nostrils, sagging jowls.	Expansion and inefficient function of aveoli. Poor resiliency of lung and diaphragm.
LARGE INTESTINE	Swelling around outside of lower lip.	Expansion of intestines, tendency towards irregularity, loose, unformed stools.
	Tightness of lower lip.	Constipation.
	Purple color of lips.	Hardness and inactivity of organ function.
	Heaviness in eyes.	Gas, heaviness in hara, unformed stools.
STOMACH	Swollen upper lip	Expanded stomach; if red, inflamed.
	Hardness and white color around border of upper lip	Expanded stomach, indigestion, chaotic eating from yin to yang.
SPLEEN/LYMPH	Swelling of temples.	Sluggishness and fatigue.
	Greenish color and/or pocked temples.	Pre-cancerous condition of the lymph system.
PANCREAS	Horizontal lines appear across the bridge of the nose.	Hyper or hypoglycemia.
	Bluish green color in diagnosis area.	Hypoglycemia, always hungry, craves sweet taste.

Cause	Personality and Postural Expression
Excess yang intake and influence, smoking.	Narrow or sunken chest, lacks aspiration.
Excess yin intake and influence, dairy foods. Milk, liquids.	Devil's advocate' personality; lack of shoulder movement when walking.
Sugar, alcohol, coffee	Meekness; doesn't look directly at people when speaking to them.
Flour products, chocolate, poor chewing, fast eating.	Goes from one project to another without completion, overly self conscious.
Excess yang animal food, salt.	Withholds emotion and expression of disagreement.
Cold producing food, liquids, drugs and medication.	Overly shy, slouches when sitting.
Poor food combinations, overeating, lack of order in eating.	Dull listless responses.
Lack of chewing, sugar and spices.	Crosses legs and bends forward when sitting.
Chronic overeating.	Stubbornness.
Gourmet food, overeating.	Overly concerned about food, eccentric tastes.
Poor quality refined and fast foods.	Lack of will, poor memory.
Excessive intake of eggs.	Irritable, overbearing, expects from others more than they are willing to give.
Excess protein.	Lacks endurance and physical strength.

Organ	Facial Appearance	Related Conditions
HEART	Red nose and face.	High blood pressure.
	Purple nose.	Low blood pressure.
	Slash mark in ear lobe and/or nasal hair.	Circulatory disorders.
SMALL INTESTINE	Swelling in central part of the lips.	Poor absorption, always hungry, fatigue.
	Horizontal lines and swelling in the center of forehead.	Stagnation and mucus clogging the intestinal function.
BLADDER	Swelling and/or wetness of upper forehead.	Organ weakness and inefficient function.
	Contraction and darkness of face around the mouth.	Frequent urination due to bladder constriction.
KIDNEY	Swollen bags under eyes.	Swollen kidneys, stones, edema.
	Purple around eyes.	Hardness of kidneys from expansion, frequent urination.
	Crows' feet (cracking horizontal lines on outside of eyes).	Tired, overworked kidneys.
	Darkness around eyes.	Frequent or infrequent urination, impotence.
LIVER	Puffy and swollen between the eyebrows.	Lack of consistent energy, loud voice.
	Tightness, contraction and vertical lines between the eyes.	Impatient, workaholic.
GALLBLADDER	Bags in upper inside corner of the eye.	Gallstones.
	Bumpy and greasy along eyebrow ridge.	Organ clogged, yellow in eye sclera.

Cause	*Personality and Postural Expression*
Animal food.	Posture emphasises chest.
Alcohol, sugar, coffee, fruit, medication.	Voice is weak, handshake is limp, expresses lack of determination.
Animal food.	Slow mind and reaction.
Flour products, refined foods, poor chewing.	Lower back is concave, timid approach.
Dairy food, saturated fats, mucus producing foods.	Bulging middle hara, "Pot belly."
Excess liquid, especially soft drinks, wine.	Incessant talking nature, nervous.
Excess salt and dry foods.	Body is tight and hard, stubborn.
Excess liquids, salt, mucus-producing foods, flour products.	Lower back does not move when walking.
Cold liquids. tropical fruit and vegetables, fruit juices. drugs.	Frozen stiff pelvic region.
Excess liquid, alcohol.	Always trying to be humorous.
Excess salt, dry and baked foods, excess sexual activity.	Uptight nature, always in a hurry. Poor sense of balance, leans forward.
Greasy, oily, fatty foods, eggs, meat, alcohol.	Sharp body movements, stands with hands on hips.
Salt and animal foods.	Demanding personality, wants things done their way.
Dairy foods and cold liquids.	General body hardness and stiffness in movement.
Dairy food, fried food and butter.	Piercing gaze and cutting expression from the eyes.

Organ	*Facial Appearance*	*Related Conditions*
OVARY TESTICLE NERVOUS SYSTEM	Yin *Sanpaku:* the eyes rise in head with white showing below and on both sides.	Organ or system weakness.
LIVER AND NERVOUS SYSTEM	Yang *Sanpaku:* the white of the eyes are visible above and on either side of the eye.	Mental problem, prone to irrational violence.
THYROID	Bulging eyes.	Hypoactivity, slow metabolism.
OVARIES	Sagging at corner of the mouth.	Weakness or removal of ovary on side of sagging.
FEMALE SEXUAL ORGANS	Area around mouth has a greenish hue or appears to be synthetic or estranged from the rest of the face.	Hysterectomy, hormone problem, sterile.
UTERUS	Crooked space under nose.	Tilted or prolapsed uterus, fibroid tumor.
PROSTATE	Swollen and hard under lower lip, in the center.	Enlarged prostate or clogged, past infection, weak erection.
	Protrusion of eyebrow ridge.	Prostate difficulty, possibly cancer.

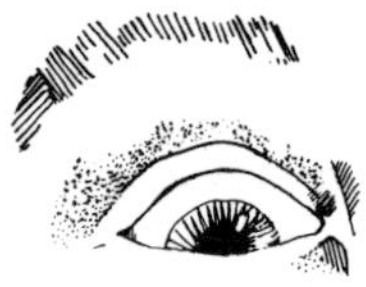

Yang Sanpaku

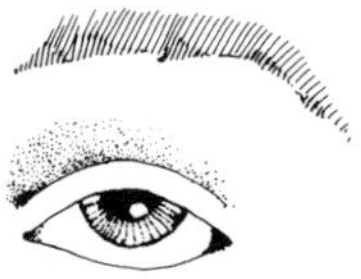

Yin Sanpaku

Cause	*Personality and Postural Expression*
Sugar, drugs, medication, soft drinks, fast foods.	Craned neck, person seems like they are melting.
Drugs, animal food, lack of whole carbohydrate, extremes of yin and yang.	Overly distracted by detail, bizarre personality.
Lack of minerals.	No sex drive or determination in life. Fear.
Dairy food, stimulants, birth control pills. Weakness due to previous removal of tonsils and gallbladder.	Aggressive, masculine nature, sharp facial lines, hard to please.
Surgery, radiation, cancer.	Narrowing of hips and loss of mass in buttocks.
Food excess of extreme yin (refined foods) or extreme yang (animal protein).	Fear of childbirth, resentment towards men, broken relationships. Sagging pelvis.
Ice cream, nuts, wine, fruit, juice, cheese.	Impatient, trouble relating to women.
Meat, eggs, cheese, ice cream.	Avoids women, attempts to dominate relationships. Stiffness in the lower back or legs.

The Facial Map

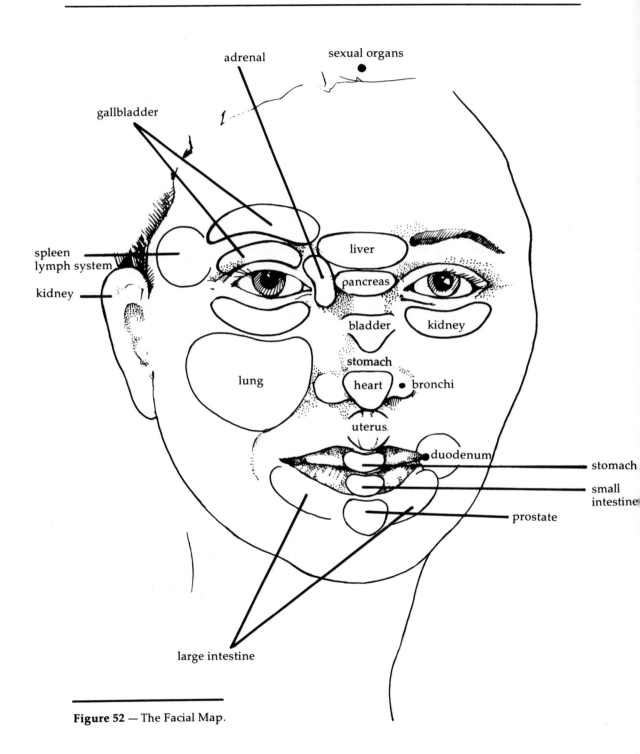

Figure 52 — The Facial Map.

Five Transformation Diagnosis

All qualities and expressions that manifest and appear in our body can be seen as extensions of the five transforming stages of energy. These energies, which are directing embryonic development, condense to create our organs and system functions as well as structures. When there is balance in an energy field, all its related functions will appear healthy. Lack of balance and/or stagnation will usually appear to some degree in most of the correlated areas in the form of functional disorder, pain or discoloration.

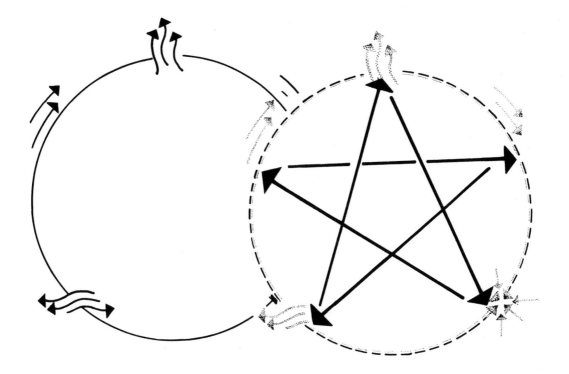

The following chart lists the different functional and structural counterparts of each energy system.

energy stage:	fire	soil
related organ:	heart/small intestine	spleen/pancreas/stomach
abnormal color:	red, pink, purple	brown, orange
sense organ:	tongue	mouth
sense:	speech	taste
voice:	laughing	sing-song
smell:	burnt	sweet
systems:	circulatory	lymph
emotional expression:		
balanced	happy and and tranquil	sympathetic, trusting, encouraging
imbalanced	excitable emotional	jealous, cynical doubtful, skeptical
tissue:	blood vessels	flesh
flower:	complexion	lips
body fluid:	sweat	saliva
taste:	bitter	sweet
time of day:	10:00 a.m.-3 p.m.	3:00 p.m.-7:00 p.m.
season:	summer	late summer
body area:	neck, left shoulder joint	knees and elbows

metal	*water*	*wood/tree*
lung/large intestine	kidney/bladder, sexual	liver/gallbladder
pale, ashen	black, blue	green, yellow
nose	ears	eyes
smell	hearing	sight
weepish, whining	groaning, gargling	shouting, sharp tone
fishy, medicated	putrid, decaying, urine	rancid
respiratory, eliminative	renal, hormone	nervous system
understanding, positive, social, enthusiastic	courageous and initiating	patient, enduring
negative, depressed, worried, territorial	fearful and anxious	impatient, frustrated, angry
skin	bones/teeth	muscles/tendon/ligaments
body hair	hair	toe nail
mucus	urine	tears
pungent	salty	sour
7:00 p.m.-12:00 a.m.	12:00 a.m.-5:00 a.m.	5:00 a.m.-10:00 a.m.
fall	winter	spring
shoulders	ankles and wrists	right shoulder joint and blades

Basic Frame Outline Diagnosis

As you work through the frame outline of your shiatsu treatment, impressions of sight and touch can be used for basic and preliminary diagnosis. If an area feels resilient this generally shows balance. Sensations like heat, cold, hardness, softness, mushiness, roughness, tenderness, or enlargement indicate unbalanced conditions. If the receiver responds with pain to the application of pressure this also indicates imbalance.

The Back

The three areas of the back show the condition of the organs and systems directly located in that region.

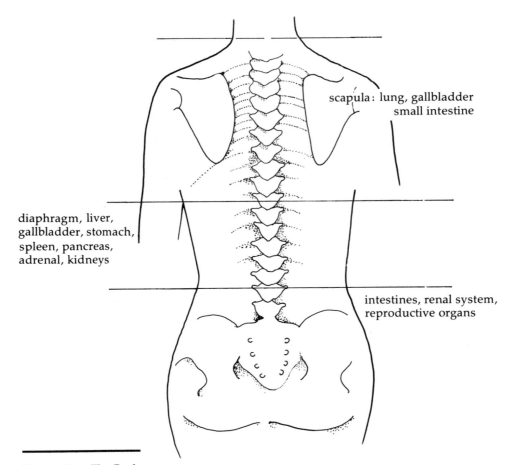

scapula: lung, gallbladder small intestine

diaphragm, liver, gallbladder, stomach, spleen, pancreas, adrenal, kidneys

intestines, renal system, reproductive organs

Figure 53 — The Back.

The Leg

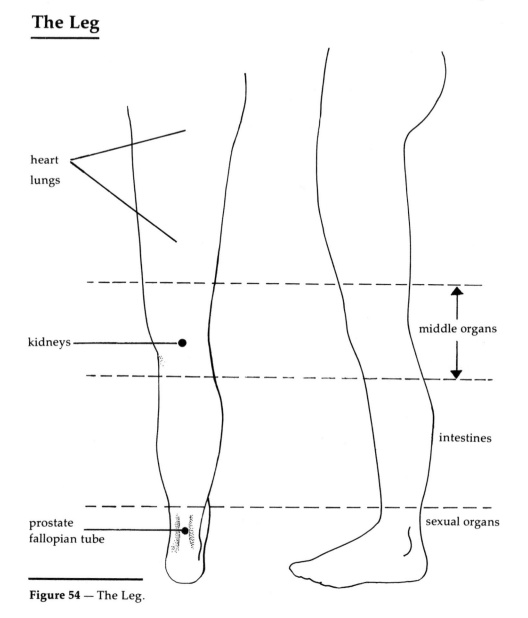

Figure 54 — The Leg.

1 The thigh is related to sexual organs.
2 The knees are related to middle organs.
   The right side: more liver/gallbladder.
   The left side: more stomach/spleen-pancreas.
   Back of knee: kidney/bladder.
3 The calf is related to intestines.
4 Ankles are related to sexual organs.
5 The Achilles tendon is related to prostate in men and the fallopian tubes in women.

The Feet

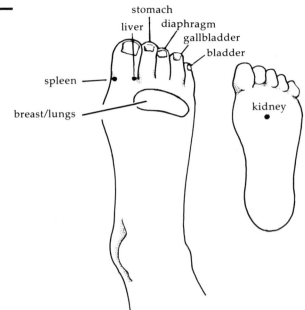

stomach
liver | diaphragm
gallbladder
bladder

spleen —•

breast/lungs

kidney
•

Figure 55 — The Feet.

1 Each toe is related to a particular energy and organ.

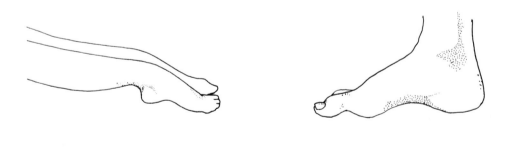

Figure 56 — Dropped Feet.   **Figure 57** — Clenched Toes.

2 Dropping foot shows lung difficulty and an overall weak condition. A person's feet drop at the time of dying. (Fig. 56)

3 Pulled back feet with clenched toes show that the liver/gallbladder has a problem. It is caused by the intake of chicken, eggs, shellfish and by fear of making change. (Fig. 57)

4 Swollen ankles and feet show kidney disorder.
5 Broken blood vessels indicate kidney disorder.
6 Purple, cold feet indicate frigidity due to ovarian stagnation in women and, in men, weak sex drive.
7 Resiliency of flesh under the large toe indicates the power of the testicles.
8 The area between the upper arches and the first flange of the toe indicates, primarily, breast for women, lung for men.

The Arm

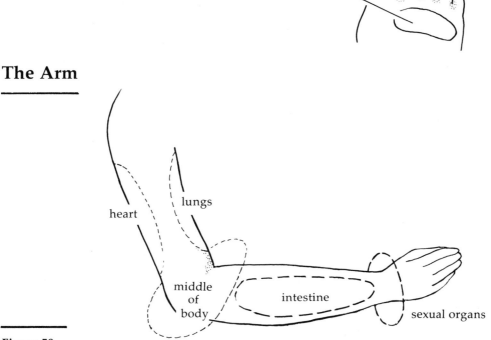

Figure 58 —

1 The upper arm shows lung and heart.
2 The elbows are related to middle organs:
    A Right side: liver/gallbladder.
    B Left side: stomach/spleen, pancreas.
3 Forearms are related to the large intestine and metabolism.
4 Wrists are related to sexual organs.
5 Along the inside middle of the forearm is related to:
    A In women: sexual function, menstrual cycle.
    B In men: lungs.
6 The inside forearm, as a whole, shows breasts.
    A A greenish, purplish hue indicates potential for cancer.
    B Fat nodules indicate the potential for cysts.

The Hands

1 Each finger is correlated with an energy system.
2 The major lines of the palm are related to the body systems.

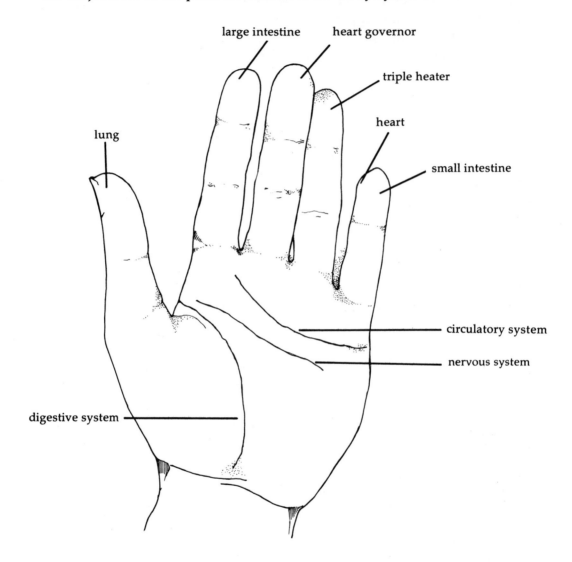

3 Puffy glazed hands indicate swollen, weak heart.
4 Hard stiff hands indicate arterial sclerosis.
5 Swollen hands with swollen finger tips indicate lung disorder.
6 Hard, cold hands show poor breathing habits, restricted circulation.
7 Blotchy red color around the heels of the hands indicates emotional difficulty.

8 The web between thumb and index finger is related to:
   A Left hand: descending colon.
   B Right hand: ascending colon.
     Greenish hue indicates potential cancer.
   C If grey in color or swollen: lungs.
9 Base of the thumb indicates lungs.
   A Grey color indicates poor oxygenation; emphysema;
     excess carbon dioxide in blood.

The Shoulders

1 The shoulders show a person's relationship with authority.
   A Left side: father or male figure.
   B Right side: mother or female figure.
   C Slumping shoulders indicate dejection, depression.
     apathy, tiredness towards life.
   D Stiff pulled-back shoulders indicate defiance, resistance,
     defensiveness.
   E Shoulder blades that protrude back indicate weak
     intestines, weak sexual organs.

2 Shoulders show lungs and intestines.
3 Right shoulder joint is related to liver and blood circulation through the liver.
4 Left shoulder joint is related to heart.

The Neck

1 The back of the neck indicates bladder, liver, gallbladder.
2 The side of the neck shows digestive tract.
3 The neck craned forward indicates:
   A Poor circulation to head.
   B Brain tires easily.
   C Organs of perception are weak and dull.
4 Stiff neck indicates rigid thinking.
5 Swollen neck with enlarged blood vessels and flush color indicates:
   A High blood pressure.
   B Suppressed anger.
   C Overly disciplined.

Appendix

The Physiology of Relaxation

Mind, Body and Spirit Connections

There is a physical mechanism and change connected with relaxation. The study of this mechanism is a major stepping stone in our shiatsu course. It is also based on the responses of the nervous system and how these responses reflect and connect the energy systems to the physical sensations with which we are more familiar. The nervous system serves as a bridge between invisible 'ki' energy and the physical manifestations of energy such as bones, muscle, tissue, and blood.

In the body, expanded energy forms such as liquids, gases and electrical impulses are more yin. Contracted, materialized or solid energy forms such as bones, muscle and tissue are more yang.

The nervous system, acting as a conduit translates what is in the energy system and over-all spirit of a person into their physical being. Thus, we can see in the physical posture the representation of the total expression of spirit, personality, psychology and emotions.*

What Happens Naturally

The nervous system has a conscious part, (the voluntary nervous system) that responds to our commands and an unconscious part, (the autonomic nervous system) that functions automatically. The autonomic nervous system triggers, coordinates, and executes all of the basic bodily functions that we tend to take for granted.

When we study the nervous system we see that amazing things happen in our bodies as a direct result of nature's process and order, which are coordinated through our energy and nervous system. Chemical reactions and transmutations of elements and compounds are occurring continuously. Matter is changing into energy and energy into matter in order to maintain our human form and to allow the body to function. Re-creating these processes is far beyond the capabilities of our present technology and is essentially irreplicable in the scientific laboratory. In the liver alone, for example, there are over one hundred chemical and energetic transmutations, such as the filtering and neutralizing of potentially harmful toxins, occuring constantly. Modern science can reproduce this type of activity only through atomic reactions that create tremendous heat and environmental disruption. On the other hand, completely safe low-heat atomic fission is pro-

---

*The word posture itself has taken on new dimensions in our modern language. Before, it was correlated mostly with physical structure. Now people are using this word, especially in corporate and organizational communication, to relay how a person feels about a situation. Thus, they are asking, "What is your posture on this proposal?" It is a very active meaning which asks, "How does your entire being align with this? How do you express yourself wholly with this situation?"

duced continuously and naturally by our biological system. Another example of the body's amazing work is the mother's production of milk after giving birth. First, the food the mother eats is broken down by chewing and through multiple actions of the digestive system. The by-product of these actions is transformed into red and white blood cells and plasma which then travel throughout the body recruiting other cells, fluids, and energies. The mother's blood then changes within the breast tissues into a liquid of totally different composition and character. By modern scientific standards these transmutations are an absolute phenomenon and are mostly unexplainable. In the body these changes, which are an activity and result of energy and its conduction systems, occur naturally without conscious effort or thought.

Para and Orthosympathetic System and Senses

The orthosympathetic branch of the autonomic nervous system is correlated more with the different experiences and expressions of tension. When overstimulated, it causes the body as a whole to close and creates resistance. This is not the type of resistance related to the prevention of sickness; rather, it is the resistance to change and adaptation that creates sickness. The parasympathetic system allows us to relax. When relaxing, the body opens and energy flows, allowing and encouraging adjustments and adaptations.*

The functioning of the para- and orthosympathetic systems is a good example of the following basic operational principle of energy:

Yang (△) at extreme of activity turns into yin (▽).
Yin (▽) at extreme of activity becomes yang (△).

Para nerves receive more of heaven's downward, inward force. They then create the opposite effect as they cause the body to open and relax. Ortho nerves, on the other hand, receive more of earth's upward, outward force, thus causing the body to tighten and close. The structure and location of the nerves are good examples of how our form and function evolve from and resemble the earth and its environment. (Fig. A1.)

---

*Actual resistance to sickness is the ability of the internal environment to adapt to the influences of external change. This enables the body to stay within the parameters of equilibrium native to the organism. Sickness originates from the body's resistance or inability to adapt and maintain balance. Even stress, which is an emotional inability to adapt, originates in accord with basic body conditions that resist change. An example of this is the body's response to refined sugar which stresses the body and with prolonged use eventually causes it to lose the ability to adapt to the extreme conditions this refined food creates. Initially minerals are borrowed from the blood, cells, and bones to neutralize these effects. In the long run however, refined sugar depletes the body of basic strengthening constituents. This creates a deep weakness that affects the total function of the body, including one's thinking, behavior and ability to operate effectively within the natural and social environments.

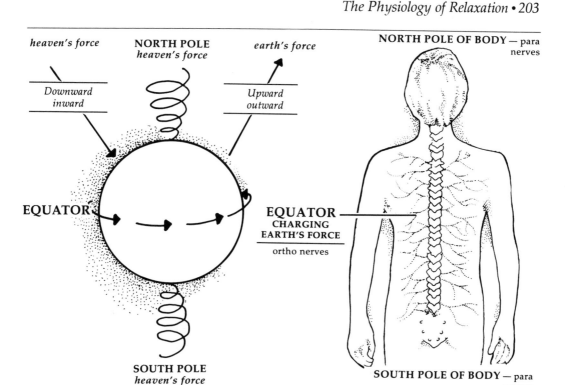

Figure A1 —

Para nerves extend from the head down and the sacrum up, imitating the earth's north and south poles where heaven's yang (△) force primarily enters our atmosphere. Ortho nerves branch out from the spine along the back. They represent the equator which most strongly generates earth's yin (▽) force.

Cooperation, Balance, and Extremes

Ideally, both branches of the autonomic nervous system operate in a cooperative relationship. Depending upon the need of function or in order to react to the environment, the energetic charges of the body will accelerate the activity of one of the branches giving it dominance over the other. Extreme conditions can develop in the body for various reasons such as dietary imbalance, emotional stress, or environment demands. Generally, inbalanced or extreme conditions will begin to create an excess, chronically overcharged ortho system along with its sensibility and correlated manifestations. If this continues over a period of time, the ortho branch of the autonomic system will begin to take control.

The para system is slightly dominant as long as conditions remain within the normal range of balance. Overall, in a healthy state the body should maintain a slightly more active charge to the para system similar to the way in which it maintains a slightly alkaline blood quality. (Fig. A2.)

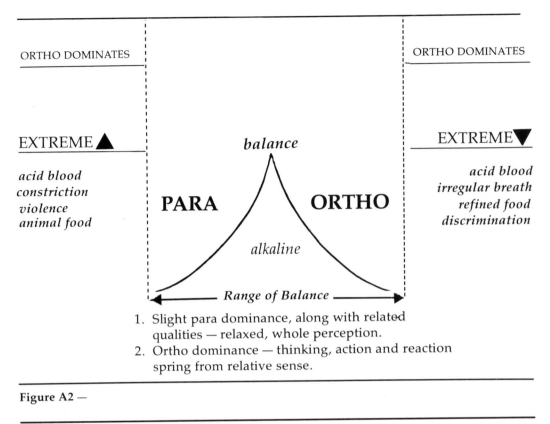

ORTHO DOMINATES

ORTHO DOMINATES

EXTREME ▲

balance

EXTREME ▼

acid blood
constriction
violence
animal food

PARA

ORTHO

acid blood
irregular breath
refined food
discrimination

alkaline

◄———— *Range of Balance* ————►

1. Slight para dominance, along with related qualities — relaxed, whole perception.
2. Ortho dominance — thinking, action and reaction spring from relative sense.

Figure A2 —

Physical Influences

The process of digestion is activated by a dominant charge in the para system. If a person is tense and the body is closed via exposure to stimulus that accelerates the ortho branch, (see Environmental Influences) digestion is inhibited. Para activates digestive secretions of the salivary glands, stomach and intestines. It charges the peristalsis of the entire digestive tract allowing the body to break down, absorb, and utilize food. Proper chewing of our food further activates the digestion by stimulating the parasympathetic related nerve plexus of the jaw joint. This stimulation triggers the secretion of digestive enzymes and signals the rest of the digestive tract into action.

Organs, muscles, and tissues are affected differently, according to their structure, by the two nervous system branches. The para system will open a tightly structured or yang (△) sphincter muscle. It also relaxes the more solid organs. For example, the heart slows down and relaxes under the influence of the parasympathetic nervous system. The orthosympathetic system, however, accelerates the heart rate. A hollow organ, yin, (▽) structure will be tightened by the para and relaxed by the ortho. When the ortho is too active the stomach cannot close to activate digestion but instead will open and relax along with the intestines. Over a period of time this can become a chronic condition contributing to constipation, diarrhea, flatulence and overeating due to poor nutrition. (Fig. A3).

	▲ *Organ or Structure*	▼ *Organ or Structure*
para	opens and relaxes	closes and tightens
ortho	closes and tightens	opens and relaxes

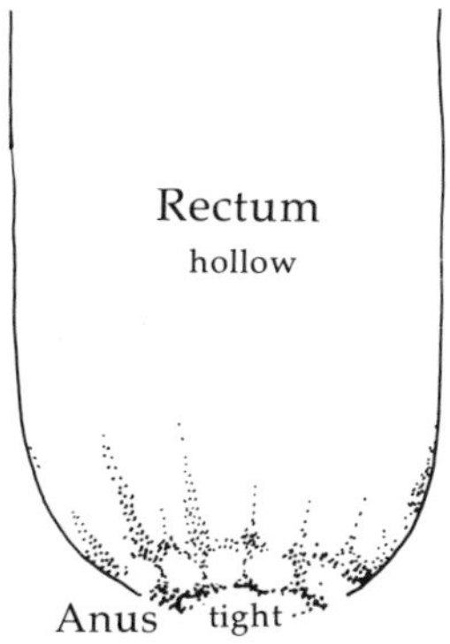

Rectum
hollow

Anus tight

Parasympathetic closes the rectum and opens the anus allowing elimination.
When relaxed it is easier to move the bowels. Ortho relaxes the rectum and closes the anus creating conditions such as constipation.

Figure A3 —

The bladder is a hollow sac and opens by a sphincter muscle. When the body relaxes (para), the bladder will close and the sphincter will open, discharging urine. In many urinary problems the orthosympathetic system is too active, constricting the opening while inhibiting the contraction of the bladder. Urination occurs frequently with very little fluid being discharged. There is a feeling of pressure due to the expanded and full bladder which does not have the ability to empty properly.

Sexual functions are also affected by these autonomic relationships. Male erection occurs as the para dilates the vascular system and allows blood to rush into the sponge-like tissues of the penis. Orgasm is triggered by the ortho charge which simultaneously constricts blood-flow through the arteries. Men who are unable to relax for various reasons may develop impotence. If the ortho is overstimulated, orgasm can occur prematurely. This is the reason traditional sexual practices have always incorporated deep relaxation as a preliminary to lovemaking. If a woman can not relax, her glands will not secrete lubricating fluid. This contributes to frigidity and inability to achieve orgasm. (Fig. A4.)

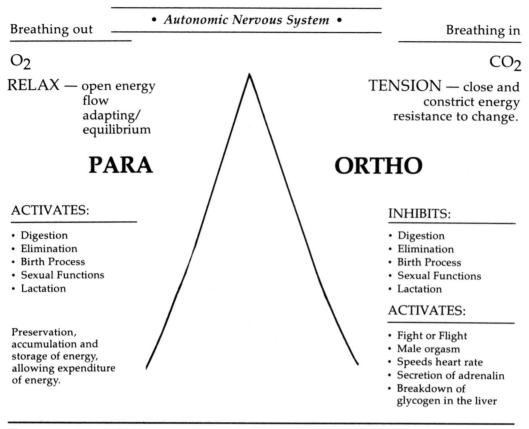

Breathing out — Breathing in

O_2

RELAX — open energy
flow
adapting/
equilibrium

PARA

ACTIVATES:

- Digestion
- Elimination
- Birth Process
- Sexual Functions
- Lactation

Preservation,
accumulation and
storage of energy,
allowing expenditure
of energy.

CO_2

TENSION — close and
constrict energy
resistance to change.

ORTHO

INHIBITS:

- Digestion
- Elimination
- Birth Process
- Sexual Functions
- Lactation

ACTIVATES:

- Fight or Flight
- Male orgasm
- Speeds heart rate
- Secretion of adrenalin
- Breakdown of
  glycogen in the liver

Figure A4 — Physical influences

Breathing

Breathing, which is a function of the senses and the energy system combined, is another activity influenced by the autonomic branches. Steady even breathing, along with the smooth intake of oxygen and complete discharge of carbon dioxide, influences the degree of balance between the two autonomic systems. Irregular or shallow breathing causes a build-up of carbon dioxide in the body contributing to an acid-blood condition which creates a state of heightened tension. These combined factors trigger over-activity of the ortho system along with many of its related conditions. An extreme alkaline condition, which is much less common, can also trigger over-activity of the same ortho system responses, causing palpitations. (Fig. A5.)

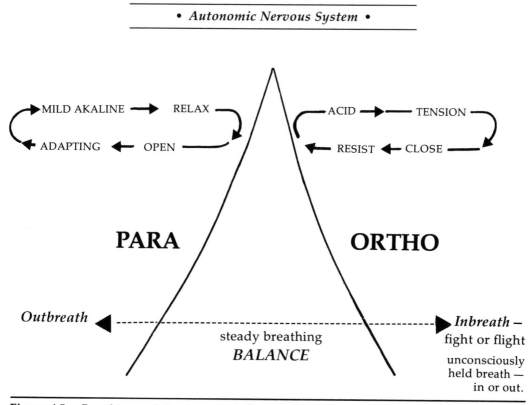

Figure A5 — Breathing and the Autonomic Nervous System

All relaxation, meditation, and spiritual development practices include breathing techniques. The effects of deep breathing and proper oxygenation stimulate the parasympathetic senses and govern the orthosympathetic senses. People always feel calm and revitalized after these practices because para action is directed toward the maintenance, accumulation, and storage of energy. The ortho activities are directed more towards the breaking down and utilization of energy by influencing the metabolism of glycogen in the liver. When ortho overrides para, energy is continuously discharged without being replenished resulting in a fatigued, burned out, depleted feeling. However when the autonomic relationship is balanced, the para is gathering energy while the ortho is directing and expending it resulting in an energized and relaxed state.

When there is too much stimulation to the para system, the excess is automatically transferred to the ortho system which handles extremes. This condition is usually induced artificially by drugs or by reactions to extreme circumstances. The result is actually a further weakening of the para system and an ineffective, further-depleting attempt by the ortho system to assume the functions of the para system. When this occurs, a person is usually experiencing a serious degenerative disease such as multiple sclerosis, Parkinson's disease, or cancer. This situation can also be created by shock from an accident or from severe burns.

Conscious holding of the breath during yoga or meditation practices nourishes the body and nervous system with oxygen and helps us gain control over some of the autonomic functions. When the breath is held in or out due to unconscious, irregular or shallow breathing, our oxygen supply is depleted to a dangerously low level. If this depletion persists over a period of time, it triggers the body's survival mechanism which functions as part of the ortho system and serves as an alarm system to get us breathing. During this process the heart speeds up and adrenalin is discharged into the bloodstream creating additional ortho-related activity.

In normal breathing or in special breathing exercises, in-breath is more related to tension, preparation, and acceleration. Out-breath is connected to relaxation, calming, and slowing down. Overall, our breathing habits affect and reflect the balance and function of the autonomic system and its related senses.

Thinking, Perception, and Behavior

The condition of the autonomic nervous system affects our physical functions and is interconnected with the orientation of all other forms of emotional, intellectual, psychological, behavioral, perceptual, and spiritual expressions. In the womb we experience almost exclusively the 'parasympathetic type sense' as we receive all stimuli as an undifferentiated unit. We begin to develop more ortho-sympathetic senses upon emerging from the womb.

Ortho sensibility is related to our conditioned responses and our ability to make sensory distinctions. It tends to pull things apart analytically making them separate and unrelated. In this mode of perception we scrutinize, discriminate, and put value comparisons on what we see. We relate to circumstances as either good or bad, and we decide what we like or dislike and want or do not want.

When the parasympathetic mode is more stimulated, we think and experience phenomena spatially, in a total perspective and in the context of wholeness. We integrate the components of our environment and perceive them as operating interdependently. We see the circumstances of success and failure, happiness and sadness, sickness and health, love and hate as two inherent sides of a single coin called the experience of life.

In the body, ortho acts as a protection response, scrutinizing and controlling stimuli until the deeper para senses can adapt to them. If the deeper para senses are unable to adapt, the surface ortho responses will act to reject the stimuli. Sustained overactive stimulation of these protection responses due to body imbalances expresses itself in accentuated imbalanced personality and behavioral traits. This creates an expression and perception of stress, defensiveness, and protectiveness. It becomes difficult to acknowledge ideas other than our own. We want things our way and feel uncomfortable in what we perceive as foreign environments. We feel difficulty, rigidity, and detachment in coping with the requirements and demands of the changing world around us.

When para functions properly it cooperates with ortho allowing us to adapt and integrate stimuli from the environment into our being. When the autonomic branches are working in harmony they create an attitude of acceptance without expectation. A balanced autonomic nervous system allows us to relax and gives us the ability to continually adapt to the constant flow of change in our surrounding universe.

As previously stated, a person functioning with a dominant ortho charge (which is typical of most people in modern society) observes things close up, picking them apart, and focusing on detail. In learning shiatsu, for example, students start by looking for points and meridians. They memorize all of the information and concepts, often overlooking the operation of the whole. In viewing a painting a person defines the brush stroke, criticizes the color scheme, and attaches to it a monetary value. A parasympathetically oriented person steps back and views the painting as a whole, sensing the spirit of the artist and feeling what is being expressed.

It is no coincidence that people who are involved with parasympathetic-stimulating activities such as yoga, meditation, and shiatsu, seem to suddenly change their ways and view of life. To those around them they seem more calm and peaceful. They are attracted to food, music, goods and environment of a more natural quality as they develop a sense of appreciation for nature. They express more joy and happiness and appear satisfied by simplicity in day to day living.

Orthosympathetic responses in balance with parasympathetic responses are a natural integrated aspect of our growth, experience, and relationships within our environment. However if these responses become a chronic syndrome we lose the wholeness and quality in our lives. We become preoccupied with the results of actions at the expense of appreciating the wealth of experience within the process. We are frustrated and impatient in 'getting there' and are unable to 'be here now.' We can see only the beauty of the flower without appreciating its relationship to the root, stem, and leaves that produce it.

Studies of science in tandem with ancient philosophy show us that everything exists and works as a whole; all phenomena are created and connected by a fabric of vibration and energy. Balance of the autonomic nervous system gives us this absolute sense and a reality of all things in nature operating together. It keeps us connected to our source and origin as we function within this relative world. (Fig. A6.)

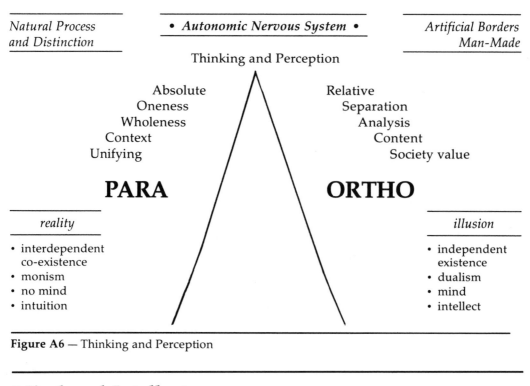

Figure A6 — Thinking and Perception

Mind and Intellect

Mind and intellect tend to work together with the orthosympathetic senses. As more and more extreme conditions develop, they produce a separating, one-sided mentality. Mind, by nature, likes to create judgement and exclusive views. This begins on the personal level and in extreme cases, extends to the social and cultural levels. This tendency is reflected in our modern economic system, current educational approach, and religious views.

Mind at an extreme, produces the small 'i', ego, or 'me' consciousness. It generates the illusion of being disconnected from others and of being in competition for survival. It creates artificial borders and territorial separation among people and countries. As a result of these extremes man has become distanced from his most primary relationship with nature as he sees himself needing to conquer his environment. In the process, he has misused and depleted our natural resources and destroyed the quality of the soil, water, air and energy sources upon which our society totally depends for sustenance.

Mind and intellect are useful tools in our enjoyment and experience of the world around us. However, they tend to create an unrealistic view of life when we choose them as our base of understanding. It is not easy for the modern educated person to realize that there is a higher, more appropriate way of knowing and perceiving. This is made available to us through what is called *"no mind"* or intuition. Intuition is related to the autonomic nervous system and requires deep strength of the parasympathetic branch.

Influences of the Environment

There are many stimuli in our modern environment that create an excessive and chronic charge to the ortho system and its related senses, weakening and immobilizing the para system and its senses.

Artificially bright atmospheres, loud noises created by machinery, ringing of the telephones, and many people talking at once, continuously alert us on a subliminal level thus creating a constant overstimulation to the ortho system. Driving, especially in traffic or at high speeds, with loud honking horns, truck noises which keep us in a state of alert, and screeching brakes, creates a defensive, tense condition and preparedness for survival. These situations cause chronic over-secretion of the adrenal glands, accelerated heart rate and digestive disorders as they are all interrelated with direct ortho stimulation and its 'fight or flight' mechanism.

Exposure to fluorescent lighting, synthetic fiber clothing, forced air heating and air conditioning, electrical appliances, and other examples of technology, continuously contribute to an imbalanced charge in the nervous system responses.

Artificial technology creates an excess of positive ionization. This interferes with the naturally balanced polarity of our internal and external electrical environments. This situation does not support the biological functions of our organic life and immobilizes our energy-gathering and storing capabilities connected with the parasympathetic nervous system.

It is interesting that, in a life-encouraging and supportive environment there is a slight dominance of positive (+) over negative (−) ions similar to the slight control of the para system and a mildly alkaline blood quality existing in healthy body conditions. Seeing the interconnectedness of these crucial balances requires that we view them from a large perspective and is a preliminary understanding of wholistic health care.

In an attempt to compensate for the lack of energetic support from the artificial environment, the body, and in particular the nervous system, depletes its energy and energy sources in its struggle to function. Energy is depleted as energy-receiving and energy-replenishing operations begin to decelerate and atrophy. This is why people working under fluorescent lights and in hermetically sealed rooms experience 'burnout' or a 'wired', hyperactive (or hyper-depressed) stressful condition. Ortho becomes hyperactive in its attempt to compensate, while para becomes weaker in its attempt to relate to the surrounding input. Ironically, most of our modern day hospitals and related health care facilities are operating in these same environments that create and sustain illness, disease and stress.

Food, Adaptation, and the Origin of Modern Conditions

Dietary practices are key factors in maintaining balance among all of the external and internal systems. Chemical and hormonal balance, nervous system balance, acid-alkaline balance, carbon dioxide and oxygen balance, and their interaction with $(-)$ and $(+)$ ion balance, along with all of the other environmental influences, are affected by the choice, quality, and preparation of our daily food. The results of our food processing (digestion, assimilation, and metabolism) influences, creates, balances and regulates the relationships of the other levels of activity with the overall condition and expression of human life. This encompasses anatomy, physiology, emotional and spiritual development, perceptions, and environment.

Whole cereal grains, beans and their products, whole unprocessed vegetables and vegetables from the sea, proportioned in accordance with our biological heritage* have always been the traditional dietary regimen for all cultures throughout history.

For thousands of years people have been motivated to eat strictly according to their common sense and intuition. As humanity moved away from this natural way of eating, modern society emerged with all of its many problems and incomplete understandings. Now, turning full circle, our contemporary scientific, medical, and governmental agencies are discovering and recommending that diets based on these traditional foods are a major factor in our physical, mental, and behavioral health.

Present day eating patterns either inadequately supply the materials needed for rebuilding and maintaining the body or over-supply the needed materials in forms which tax or obstruct the utilizing systems. A diet consisting of heavy animal foods, high cholesterol, saturated fats, and refined, devitalized food is now being linked to a myriad of degenerative and communicable diseases. As time passes, modern science will discover that all of the epidemic diseases now plaguing modern society are completely preventable simply by consuming a proper diet.

Knowing how diet affects our body is the key to understanding how we have chronically over-stimulated the orthosympathetic system and its related expressions.

---

*See Book of Macrobiotics by Michio Kushi, Japan Publications.

Animal foods create an excessively contracting (△) yang tendency in the body constricting the flow of energy and body fluids such as blood. During the digestive, assimilative, and metabolic processes, animal foods leave toxic by-products throughout the body. Indigestible unusable fats and cholesterol clog the body on all levels from cell to organ to responses and thinking. Overall they create a condition of struggle so that ortho-related survival mechanisms become more and more prominent. An additional problem resulting from the consumption of animal food is the acidic blood quality it helps to create, constantly activating the ortho-related conditions.

Refined, devitalized and chemicalized foods create an extreme (▽) yin or expanding tendency in the body that cannot support the flow and conduction of energies required by the body and its functions. As a result of eating these foods regularly, our overall strength and resilience is diminished at all levels from the cell walls to our capacity to adjust in day to day life. These foods seriously breakdown and degenerate the strength and constitution of our organs and devitalize our body tissues and fluids. Refined, processed foods create excess mucus which has a clogging effect, and in a similar way to their yang (△) counterparts on the other extreme, create acidic blood.

Whole food products, on the other hand, harmonize completely with the digestive, absorptive and metabolic processes and leave no toxic residues. Because of the compatibility of cereal grains with the complex carbohydrate-to-energy conversion capabilities of the digestive tract, these foods deliver a steady supply of energy with practically no waste. Grains and beans, particularly fermented soybean products, provide the body with easily convertible proteins for the rebuilding of cells, tissues, and muscles. They leave none of the poisonous ammonia or acidic wastes, the by-product of animal food, to load the kidneys. Researchers are now connecting the presence of animal food residue in the body with the formation of tumors and cancer cells.

Whole carbohydrates, an integral part of unprocessed cereal grains, are converted in the body to compounds that stimulate the functions of our brain. Incomplete, processed carbohydrates (refined sugar, honey, corn syrup, etc.) are unable to supply the proper building materials for these compounds. This deficiency can lead to learning disability and poor memory as well as temperament/behavioral problems.

Diet holds a key position in maintaining balance in body, mind and spirit. It is a unique influence in that we can create and control it completely by our own choice and free will. (Fig. A7.)

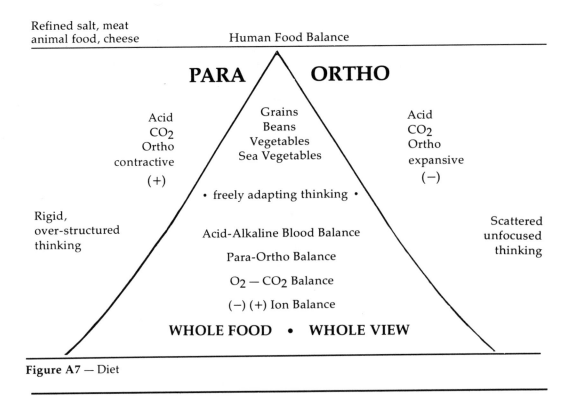

Refined salt, meat
animal food, cheese

Human Food Balance

PARA / **ORTHO**

Acid
CO_2
Ortho
contractive
$(+)$

Grains
Beans
Vegetables
Sea Vegetables

Acid
CO_2
Ortho
expansive
$(-)$

• freely adapting thinking •

Rigid,
over-structured
thinking

Scattered
unfocused
thinking

Acid-Alkaline Blood Balance

Para-Ortho Balance

$O_2 - CO_2$ Balance

$(-)$ $(+)$ Ion Balance

WHOLE FOOD • **WHOLE VIEW**

Figure A7 — Diet

Macrobiotic Standard Diet Chart

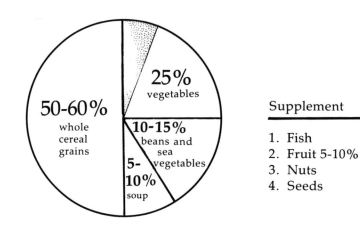

50-60%
whole
cereal
grains

25%
vegetables

10-15%
beans and
sea
vegetables

5-10%
soup

Supplement

1. Fish
2. Fruit 5-10%
3. Nuts
4. Seeds

Figure A8 — Standard Macrobiotic Diet Chart.

The standard macrobiotic diet represents the requirements for the average human constitution. Variations and adjustments need to be considered depending on individual qualities. (See Book of Macrobiotics by Michio Kushi.)

Conclusion

Through proper application of shiatsu we can encourage a deep stimulation of the parasympathetic system and induce a balancing of the orthosympathetic system. This occurs as a natural result of harmonizing the body's basic energy flows. Some recipients may experience these changes on a subliminal level only, while others are able to identify them clearly. In either case these basic energetic alignments will seek to penetrate all other levels of being, from structural to spiritual. In the time following treatment the person will begin seeking the appropriate methods or channels, such as diet, exercise and therapy, to allow this balancing of the various levels to happen.

Index